In Praise of Gina

Gina's 'Contented Little Baby' routines are based upon many years of experience and have stood the test of time. Her writings contain the wisdom of common sense and experience. Being a mother and being a father are huge steps. Whilst challenging, you will find caring for your baby one of the best experiences of your life. Gina's work will help guide you to a happier outcome and be a positive contribution to your journey.

Dr Brian Symons, The Baby Sleep Doctor

'Thank you so much, Gina Ford. You and your books are truly heaven sent.'

'Without your books I do not know what I would have done. Your advice has meant that I have a fantastic, happy little boy and I actually look forward to the next challenge he may bring as I know where the answer to any problem lies!'

'I would like to express my gratitude for your book. It has been an absolute saviour and my best friend since I started my little boy on your routine when he was 10 weeks old. He is nearly nine months old now and everyone always says of him "What a happy contented little baby!"'

'From day one of Daisy's return home from hospital we put her into Gina's routine and have never looked back. Everyone comments on Daisy and what an unbelievably happy and contented baby she is ... Thank you, Gina, for your books and the enjoyment and confidence they have given us.'

'Gina transformed our son into the happiest, "easiest" baby, that we could have wished for. Her knowledge and professionalism is astounding; she has answers to every question – and they really work.'

'My friends tell me that it is not "normal" for a baby to be as happy and well-behaved as my daughter. It certainly seems to be normal for "Gina's babies".'

'We can't recommend her highly enough to any prospective parents. We found her invaluable, and I have much to thank her for – setting us on the right path to understanding our baby's needs and being confident parents, as well as giving our son the best start in life he could get.'

To my beloved mother and best friend in blessed remembrance of all her wisdom, the very special love, support and encouragement she always gave me and whose wonderful smile and sparkling eyes could turn a rainy day into sunshine.

The New Contented Little Baby Book

The secret to calm and confident parenting

Gina Ford

Vermilion
LONDON

29

Vermilion, an imprint of Ebury Publishing,
20 Vauxhall Bridge Road,
London SW1V 2SA

Vermilion is part of the Penguin Random House group of companies whose
addresses can be found at global.penguinrandomhouse.com

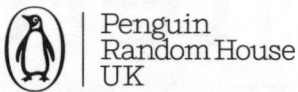

Penguin
Random House
UK

Copyright © Gina Ford 1999, 2002, 2006, 2017

Gina Ford has asserted her right to be identified as the author of this work in
accordance with the Copyright, Designs and Patents Act 1988.

www.penguin.co.uk

A CIP catalogue record for this book is available from the British Library

ISBN 9780091912697

Typeset in India by Integra Software Services Pvt. Ltd, Pondicherry

Printed and bound in Great Britain by Clays Ltd, Elcograf S.p.A.

Penguin Random House is committed to a sustainable future for our
business, our readers and our planet. This book is made from Forest
Stewardship Council® certified paper.

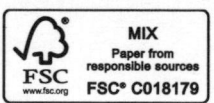

Contents

Acknowledgements — *xi*
Foreword — *xiii*
Introduction — *xvi*

1. Preparation for the Birth — 1
The nursery — 3
Baby equipment — 10
Equipment needed for breast-feeding — 18
Equipment needed for bottle-feeding — 21
Clothes for the newborn — 23
Your baby's laundry — 29

2. Why Follow a Routine? — 32
Why the CLB routines are different — 33
Benefits for your baby — 34
Benefits for you — 35
Other approaches — 36
Your questions answered — 41

3. Milk Feeding in the First Year — 54
Why breast-feeding goes wrong — 55
Milk production — 57
My methods for successful breast-feeding — 61
Expressing — 64
Milk oversupply — 67
Breast-feeding and returning to work — 69
Weaning your baby from the breast to the bottle — 71

Bottle-feeding	73
Establishing bottle-feeding	76
Formula: over-feeding	83
Giving water to babies under 6 months	83
Diluting feeds	84
Your questions answered	85
4. Understanding Your Baby's Sleep	**91**
Sleep and demand-feeding	94
Sleep rhythms	96
The bedtime routine	97
Early-morning waking	100
Your questions answered	103
5. Establishing the Contented Little Baby Routines	**108**
Feeding	108
Sleeping	110
Playing	112
Cuddling	113
Structuring the milk feeds during the first year	114
Understanding the routines for feeding	116
Structuring daytime sleep during the first year	131
Understanding the sleeping routine	133
Adjusting the routines	146
Adjusting the routine for nursery	148
Adjusting the routine for daytime outings	150
Adjusting the routines for holidays	157
Guide to sleep required during the first year	162
Important recommendations	162
6. Weeks One to Two	**164**
Starting the routine	164
Routine – one to two weeks	166

Changes to be made during the one- to two-week routine   172
Moving on to the two- to four-week routine   174

7. Weeks Two to Four   176
Routine – two to four weeks   176
Changes to be made during the two-
    to four-week routine   182

8. Weeks Four to Six   188
Routine – four to six weeks   188
Changes to be made during the four-
    to six-week routine   194

9. Weeks Six to Eight   200
Routine – six to eight weeks   200
Changes to be made during the six-
    to eight-week routine   207

10. Weeks Eight to Twelve   212
Routine – eight to twelve weeks   212
Changes to be made during the eight-
    to twelve-week routine   217
Moving on to the three- to four-month routine   220

11. Months Three to Four   221
Routine – three to four months   221
Changes to be made during the three-
    to four-month routine   225

12. Months Four to Six   231
Routine – four to six months   231
Changes to be made during the four-
    to six-month routine   235

13. Months Six to Nine   **240**
Routine – six to nine months   240
Changes to be made during the six-
to nine-month routine   244

14. Months Nine to Twelve   **249**
Routine – nine to twelve months   249
Changes to be made during the nine- to twelve-
month routine   253
Cutting out the morning nap   254

15. Introducing Solid Food   **257**
Weaning your baby   257
Foods to be avoided   260
Preparing and cooking food for your baby   262
Early weaning   264
First stage: six to seven months   267
Second stage: seven to nine months   274
Third stage: nine to twelve months   279
Your questions answered   284

16. Problem-Solving in the First Year   **291**
General problems   291
Any baby bringing up an entire feed twice in a
row should be seen by a doctor immediately   302
Common feeding problems   311
Tongue tie   332
Common sleeping problems   334
Golden rules   355
Appendix: 359
The Lullaby Trust Advice to Reduce
the Risk of Cot Death   359

Contents

Useful Addresses 361

Further Reading 364

Contentedbaby.com 366

Index 367

Acknowledgements

I would like to say a huge thank you to all the families I have worked with around the world for having so much trust and faith in my methods, and for the constant feedback that you have given me over the years as your babies have been growing up.

My publisher has also continued to give me the most enormous support and guidance, as has former publisher Fiona MacIntyre, present publisher Rebecca Smart, editors Katy Denny, Sam Jackson, Emma Owen, Imogen Fortes, Cindy Chan, and Louise Coe and the rest of the team at Penguin Random House. I owe them all a huge debt of gratitude for having such faith in my methods and encouraging my career as an author.

A very special thank you to the contentedbaby.com team, editor Kate Brian, Sofiah Macleod, Alison Jermyn and Christel Davidson, for all their wonderful work on the website and also their constant support and encouragement with the writing of my books. Also to Rory Jenkins of Embado.com, whose technical skills have helped create an amazing website which reaches parents across five continents.

Finally, I would like to say thank you to the thousands of parents whom I have worked with through my consultancy service over the last 18 years. Your feedback of how the CLB routines have worked for you has helped me hugely with the revision of this book, and your loving supportive messages mean more than you will ever know. Special love and thanks to you all and to your contented babies.

Foreword

When *The Contented Little Baby Book* was first published in 1999 I was so impressed that at long last someone was offering parents step by step guidelines to help with the practicalities of looking after their babies rather than telling them to just rely on their instincts and intuition. Since then I have witnessed first-hand how Gina's routines have been a lifeline to so many parents and it gives me great pleasure to write this foreword.

Having spent over 30 years working with mothers and babies, I see how often parents are subjected to conflicting advice, which can leave them confused and anxious. Everyone seems to have an opinion on how best to raise a baby with even the experts failing to agree on basic advice, such as feeding on demand versus routine and how to breast-feed successfully. Amidst all this confusion, the one thing that stands out to me is that establishing a degree of routine in the day leads to more settled babies and calmer, more confident parents.

Throughout this book Gina gives clear guidelines to help parents establish routines that you can take one day at a time and over the weeks will change with your baby's needs. She explains why it is important to anticipate when your baby will be tired or hungry so that he or she never has to cry to get attention or to tell you that something is wrong, Gina also offers invaluable trouble-shooting advice and explains how to adapt her routines to meet the individual requirements of your baby.

If you follow even half of the advice contained in this book, you will be well on track to having a very contented baby and being a happy and confident new parent.

Clare Byam-Cook SRN, SCM
Author of *What to Expect when You're Breast-feeding...*
and What if You Can't?

Introduction

The Contented Little Baby Book (first published in 1999), was based on my personal experiences of working and living with over 300 babies and their families in many different parts of the world. It became a bestseller and has been used, and continues to be used, by millions of families across five continents. The popularity of my advice, and loyal support of the book's followers, is testimony that babies can and do thrive very successfully on routines. Unlike the old-fashioned and inflexible four-hourly routines, my routines are based upon a baby's natural feeding and sleeping rhythms, ensuring that a baby's needs are met before he gets distressed or overtired. Most importantly, the routines can be adapted to suit the individual needs of each baby; from extensive experience, I know that all babies are different.

In the time since my first book was published, I have communicated with thousands of parents as a result of my consultancy work and through the Contented Baby website, contentedbaby.com. This regular and direct contact has enabled me to obtain useful feedback from parents on the Contented Little Baby (CLB) routines, which in turn has inspired me to fully revise and update my original book. The CLB routines and my core philosophy remain the same, but my advice has been expanded in response to this valuable feedback, and adapted to today's circumstances.

I am confident that this revised book will be even better at teaching you how to recognise the difference between hunger and tiredness, how to establish good feeding and sleeping patterns and how to meet all of your precious baby's needs. With help from this totally revised version of *The New Contented Little Baby Book*, becoming a parent should be a happy and deeply satisfying experience for both you and your baby. The CLB routines have worked for many millions of parents and their contented babies, and they can work for you, too.

Gina Ford

Gina Ford Problem Solving Consultancy

Although I no longer visit parents in their homes, I am still very involved with parents on a daily basis via my baby and toddler problem solving consultancy. If you would like personal one-to-one help with establishing a routine for your baby or are experiencing feeding, sleeping or behavioural problems with your baby or toddler, please email cbc@contentedbaby.com for details of the various types of consultations I can offer.

1

Preparation for the Birth

When one talks of preparing for the birth, the first things that spring to mind are antenatal care and decorating the nursery. Both are important in their own ways. Antenatal care is of the utmost importance for a healthy pregnancy and helps to prepare you for the birth, and decorating the nursery for the new arrival is fun. While many of the antenatal classes on offer do give some advice on what is ahead after the birth, they often focus on the birth itself and overlook very practical tips, which, if offered early enough, could save parents hours of time and stress after their baby is born.

If you follow my routines from day one you should be fortunate enough to have a contented and happy baby, with some time for yourself. However, as you will see from my routines and charts, spare time is extremely limited (and, believe me, parents who are not following a routine have even less spare time). In this short amount of time, unless you have hired help, you will have to fit in the cooking of meals, shopping, laundry, etc. By doing the following things before the baby is born you will gain many hours of free time after the birth.

- Order all your nursery equipment well in advance. Cots can sometimes take up to 12 weeks to be delivered and there are many advantages in having the big cot from the beginning (see page 4).

- Have all the bed linen, muslins and towels washed and ready for use. Make up the cot, Moses basket and pram. Prepare everything in the nursery so it is at hand the minute you get home from the hospital.

- Have the following baby essentials in stock: cotton wool, baby oil, nappies, nappy and moisturising creams, baby wipes, soft sponges, baby brush, bath oil and baby shampoo.

- Check that all the electrical equipment is working properly. Learn how the steriliser works and how to put together the feeding bottles.

- Arrange a section of work-top in the kitchen where preparation and sterilisation can be done. Ideally, it should be directly below a cupboard where all the baby's feeding equipment can be stored.

- Stock up on soap powder, cleaning materials and enough kitchen and toilet rolls to last at least six weeks.

- Prepare and freeze a large selection of healthy home-made meals for you and your husband/partner. If you are planning to breast-feed you should avoid the shop-bought ones that are full of additives and preservatives.

- Stock up on extra dry goods such as tea, coffee, biscuits, etc.; it is inevitable that you will have extra visitors during the first month, and supplies will soon go down.

- Purchase birthday gifts and cards for any forthcoming birthdays. Also have a good selection of thank you cards ready to send for all the gifts you will receive.

- Get up to date with any odd jobs that need to be done in the house or garden. The last thing you need once the baby has arrived is the hassle of workmen to-ing and fro-ing.

- If you are planning to breast-feed, book your electric expressing machine well in advance; they are in big demand! Ask your midwife for advice on how to do this.

The nursery

Like most parents, you will probably have your baby sleeping in your room with you during the night. The current advice from The Lullaby Trust (formerly FSID) and the Department of Health is that your baby should sleep in the same room as you for all sleeps until he is six months old (see page 162). However, I still believe it is important to have the nursery ready on your return from hospital. All too often a mother will ring me up in a complete panic asking for advice on how to get an older baby used to their own room.

From the very beginning, you should use the nursery as much as possible for nappy changing, feeding and some quiet play. By getting your baby used to his room from the beginning, he will very quickly enjoy being there and see it as a peaceful haven. When babies are very small, especially if they have become overtired and overstimulated, it is really useful to have a quiet, comfortable room where they can be taken to wind-down. Using your baby's nursery for this purpose in the early days will help him to make the transition from sleeping in the same room as you to sleeping in his own room, once he reaches six months.

Decoration

It is not essential to spend a fortune on decorating and furnishing the baby's room. A room with walls, windows and bed linen covered in teddy bears soon becomes very boring. Plain walls can easily be brightened up with a colourful frieze or stickers, and perhaps a matching pelmet and tie-backs; this makes it easy to adapt the room as the baby grows, but avoids the need to redecorate totally. Another very cost-effective and fun way to liven up the room is to use sheets of children's wrapping paper as posters, which are bright and colourful and can be changed frequently.

The cot

Most baby books advise that in the early days a cot is not necessary, as babies are happier in a Moses basket or small crib. While it may seem a more practical solution when moving your baby from room to room with you (see page 162 for current advice), I am not convinced babies are happier or sleep better in these. As your baby will need to get used to sleeping where you are until he is six months old, it is a better option to have a pram with a firm mattress made up for him in the room you are in that he will use for the duration of this period. It is still important to get babies to use their big cot from day one. I would recommend you allow your baby to have some playtime in his big cot with you in the room. By doing this, I never encountered a problem when they outgrew their Moses basket and started to sleep the whole night in their big cot in the nursery.

When choosing a cot, it is important to remember that it will be your baby's bed for at least two or three years and should therefore be sturdy enough to withstand a bouncing toddler. Even very young babies will eventually move around their cots. I would suggest choosing a design with flat spars instead of round ones, as pressing the head against a round spar could be quite painful for a young baby. Cot bumpers are not advised for babies less than one year old, as they can end up sleeping with their heads pressed up against the bumpers. Because body heat escapes through the top of the head, blocking it off increases the risk of overheating. This is thought to be a contributing factor in cot death.

Other points to bear in mind when choosing cots are:

- Look for two or three different base-height levels.

- The cot should be large enough to accommodate a two-year-old child comfortably.

- All cots must comply with the recommendations set out by the British Standards Institute, Number BS1753. Spars must be no less than 2.5cm (1in) and no more than 6cm (2½ in) apart. When the mattress is at its lowest position, the maximum distance between that and the cot top should be no more than 65cm (26in). There should be a gap of no more than 4cm (1½ in) around the edge of the mattress.

- Buy the best possible mattresses that you can afford. I have found that foam mattresses tend to sink in the middle within a few months. The type I have found to give the best support for growing babies is a 'natural cotton spring interior' type. All mattresses must comply with Safety Standards Numbers BS1877 and BS7177.

Bedding for the cot

Everything should be 100 per cent white cotton so that it can be washed on a hot wash along with the baby's night clothes. Due to the risk of overheating or smothering, quilts, duvets, pillows and baby nests are not recommended for babies under one year old. If you want a pretty matching top cover for your baby's cot, make sure it is 100 per cent cotton and not quilted with a nylon filling. For parents who are handy with a sewing machine, a considerable amount of money can be saved by making flat sheets and draw sheets out of a large cotton double-bed sheet.

Making up the cot

(a) Remove mattress and lay a sheet, and, depending on the time of year, possibly blanket lengthways across the width at the base of the cot.

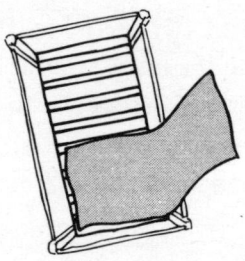

(b) Replace mattress and cover with bottom sheet.

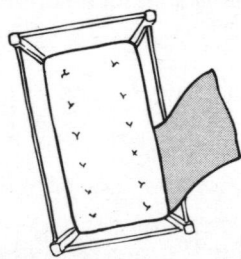

(c) Bring the covers over the top of the mattress and tuck in at least 15cm (6ins) underneath at the bottom and at the front side of the cot. Remember to leave enough untucked so that you can place baby in the cot.

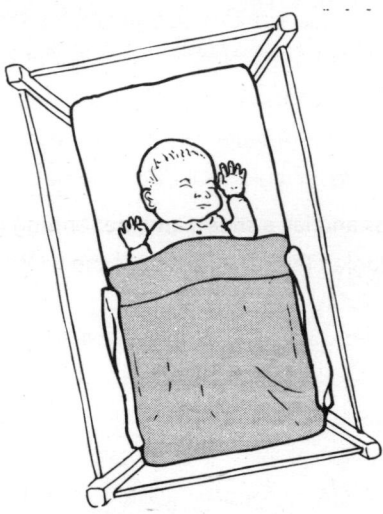

(d) When you have placed baby in the cot, ensuring that his feet are near the bottom of the cot, you should then tuck the remainder of the covers 15cm (6ins) well under the mattress.

(e) Push a small, rolled up towel down either side between the cot mattress and spars to ensure the baby cannot kick the covers off or work their way loose.

You will need the following bedding:

- Three stretch-cotton fitted bottom sheets. Choose the soft jersey-type cotton rather than the towelling type, which can very quickly become rough and worn-looking.

- Three flat, smooth cotton top sheets. Avoid flannelette, which gives off too much fluff for young babies; this can obstruct the nose and cause breathing problems.

- Three cotton, close-weave cellular blankets, plus one wool blanket for very cold nights.

- Draw sheets – six flat, smooth cotton pram sheets. These are small sheets that are used for prams and Moses baskets, which you should put across the head end of the bottom sheet. This eliminates the need to remake the whole cot in the middle of the night or during naps, should your baby dribble or his nappy leak.

Changing station

The most practical changing station is a long unit, containing drawers and a cupboard. The top should be long enough to hold both the changing mat and the top-and-tail bowl. The drawers can be used to store nightwear, underwear and muslins, and the cupboard can hold larger items, such as nappy packs.

Wardrobe

A fitted wardrobe is a very good investment for your nursery as it enables you to keep the baby's clothes tidy and crease-free, and it will also provide valuable storage space for the many pieces of equipment that you will accumulate. If a fitted wardrobe is out of the question, try to purchase a free-standing version.

Chair

It is essential, no matter how small your baby's room is, that you try to fit in a chair. A really sturdy comfortable chair is an absolute priority. A small two-seater bed-settee is a good choice as it can be used for both feeding and for sleeping in the baby's room. If space is limited, then choose a chair with a straight back. It should be wide enough to allow room for you and your baby as he grows and, ideally, the arms should be wide enough to support you while breast-feeding. I would resist the temptation to buy a rocking chair, which is often sold as a nursing chair. These can prove to be dangerous as the baby becomes more mobile and may attempt to pull himself up by holding on to the chair, which will move and could send him toppling over. In the early days it can also be tempting to settle your baby by rocking him to sleep, but this is one of the main causes of a baby developing poor sleeping habits.

Curtains

Curtains should be full-length and fully lined with blackout lining (see Useful Addresses on page 361). Fix them to a track that fits flush along the top of the window. Ideally, they should have a deep matching pelmet, which is also lined with blackout lining. There should be no gaps between the sides of the curtains and the window frame; even the smallest chink of light can be enough to wake your baby earlier than 7am. For the same reason, curtain poles should be avoided as the light streams through the gap at the top. As your baby gets older, he may not settle back to sleep if woken by early morning sun in the summer, or streetlights.

When the lights are off and the curtains are closed, it should be so dark that you are unable to see your partner standing at the other side of the room. Research has shown that the chemicals in the brain alter in the dark, conditioning the body for sleep.

Carpeting

A fully fitted carpet is preferable to rugs, which have the potential for tripping on when you are attending to your baby in dim light. Choose a carpet that is treated with a stain-guard, and avoid very dark or bright colours, as they tend to show the dirt more easily.

Lighting

If the main light in the nursery is not already fitted with a dimmer switch, it would be worthwhile changing it. In the early days, dimming the lights when settling the baby is a good association signal. If you are on a limited budget, purchase one of the small plug-in night-lights that fit into any normal 13-amp electrical socket.

Baby equipment

Moses basket or small crib

As I mentioned earlier, a Moses basket is not really essential. Even the cheapest of Moses baskets and a stand can cost between £30–45, which is quite a lot of money for something unessential that your baby will outgrow within six weeks. However, if you live in a very large house or plan to travel in the first few weeks, it may be useful. If your budget is limited, try to borrow one from a friend and buy a new mattress.

A crib is a small version of a big cot. Certainly, it is longer than a Moses basket, but not really any more practical. Because we now put our babies to sleep on their backs, these narrow cribs create a problem for small babies. They can wake themselves up several times a night because the cribs are not wide enough for them to sleep with their arms stretched out fully, and they get their hands caught between the spars.

If you do decide to use either of the above for a short period, you will need the following bedding:

- Three fixed, stretch-cotton bottom sheets. Choose the soft, smooth jersey-type cotton.
- Six flat smooth cotton pram sheets, to be used as top sheets and later as draw sheets on the big cot.

- Three cotton, cellular close-weave pram blankets.

- A dozen muslins to be placed across the top of the basket or crib to catch dribbles.

By three months the majority of babies have grown out of a Moses basket or a small crib. As it is recommended that you have your baby sleep in your room for at least the first six months, you will then be faced with a problem if your baby's cot cannot fit in your bedroom. In this case I would recommend that you invest in a compact second cot – it is possible to get one quite cheaply. Although it is an extra expense it is well worth it, and it can always be passed on for use at a grandparents' house for when you visit.

Pram

The traditional pram is very expensive and not really appropriate to modern-day living. Most parents find it more practical to choose one of the other smaller types of transport available now. When choosing a pram, carry-cot or buggy, it is important to take into consideration the fact that, according to The Lullaby Trust guidelines, you will keep your baby with you at all sleep times during the day until he is six months. It is important to take into consideration where you live and your lifestyle. A popular choice with parents is a 'three-in-one', which is a transporter that can be used with a carry-cot in the early days and later with a buggy-type seat. This can be a very good choice if you live in a quieter area and can walk to the local shops. If you have to drive to the nearest shops, it is important to choose a buggy that is easy to put up and down and not too heavy for constant lifting in and out of the car boot. There are now some very lightweight buggies on the market that recline flat for a newborn baby, and come with hood and apron to give the baby some protection in cold weather.

The third choice is a heavier-weight version of the light buggy; it also reclines flat for a newborn and usually comes with a mattress. If you are likely to be using your pram or buggy in a town area, or in shops with narrow spaces (for example, aisles in supermarkets), swivel wheels are a godsend. They make turning the buggy or pram round corners effortless compared to those with set wheels. Whichever type you choose, you should practise putting it up and down several times, and try lifting it on to a surface in the shop to get an idea of how easy it is going to be to lift into the boot. The following guidelines should also be followed when purchasing a pram, carry-cot or buggy:

- It should be fitted with good strong safety straps that go over the baby's shoulders as well as around the waist, and have an easy-to-operate brake.

- Make sure it has a hood and apron to protect the baby in colder weather.

- Buy all the extras at the same time: sun canopy, rain cover, cosytoes cover, head support cushion and shopping tray or bag. Models often change in design and sometimes dimension, and if you wait till the following season, the items you require might not fit or match.

- Try pushing it around the shop to check if the handle height is a comfortable level; also observe how easy it is to get in and out of doorways and round corners.

Car seat

You will need to have a car seat to bring your baby home from hospital. A midwife often accompanies parents to the car to check that all is in order as mother and baby are discharged. A baby car seat should always be used, even on short journeys. However, new research from the University of Bristol has shown that newborn infants may be at risk of breathing difficulties if left in car safety seats for long periods, particularly when travelling. The Lullaby Trust recommends 'parents avoid driving long distances without a break. However, avoiding the risk of injury due to a road traffic accident is paramount and fitted car seats should always be used to transport babies and toddlers.' Never be tempted to travel holding your baby in your arms as, in the event of a collision or emergency stop, it would be impossible to keep hold of your baby. Car seats should not be fitted to the front passenger seat if the car has airbags, unless these have been adequately disabled. In general, choose the best you can afford, and preferably ones that come with clear fitting instructions.

Other things to look for include:

- A seat with large side wings, which offer more protection in a side-impact collision.

- A one-pull harness, which will make it much easier to adjust the seat to your baby's clothing.

- The buckle should be easy to open and close, but not easy enough for a child to open.

- The availability of extra accessories, such as a head support pillow or replacement cover.

Baby bath

A baby bath is another item that is not essential. Like the Moses basket, babies outgrow the small bath very quickly. A newborn baby can be bathed in the hand basin to begin with, or even in a big bath using one of the several types of bath seats that are available for tiny babies. These allow the baby to lie, supported and on a slight slope, leaving the mother with both hands free to wash the baby.

If you would feel more confident with a special baby bath, the one I would recommend is designed to fit across a big bath.

It makes filling and emptying much easier, unlike the traditional baby bath that sits on a stand, and has to be filled and emptied using a bucket. Another design is a bath that is incorporated in a changing station. I have found these totally impractical because, as you lift the baby out of the bath, you have to manoeuvre the lid, which doubles as the changing table, down over the top of the bath before you can put the baby on it to dry and dress him. They are also very difficult to empty; I found I always had to tip the whole thing on its side to drain the water out completely. This usually ended up with all the items stored below toppling out on to the floor. These bath/changing stations are very expensive and I would discourage anyone from buying them.

Changing mat

It is worthwhile buying two changing mats. Choose easy-clean plastic with well-padded sides. In the early days it is best to lay a hand towel on the top, as very young babies hate to be laid down on anything cold.

Choosing a baby monitor

Once your baby is old enough to sleep in his own room most parents find a baby monitor reassuring. There is a huge choice on the market these days, from a simple monitor that enables you to listen to your baby whilst he is in another room, to ones that allow you to not only listen to your baby, but with the use of a camera you can also see what he doing. Some of the latest designs come with an app that allows you to check on your baby via your phone, wherever you are in the house and even if you are out for the evening and miles away. I think that it is worthwhile putting some effort into researching what is out there and reading the reviews from other parents before you make your decision which one to buy. I have found that most parents opt for a digital monitor with a camera that allows them to check if your baby is asleep or awake, which is very helpful with older babies who do not necessarily make a noise when they wake. Having an idea of the babies waking time can help determine what time they will need their next nap. I would also recommend a monitor with a two-way talk function, as it can be really helpful with a toddler who is going through a stage of being unsettled in the night, as you can reassure him via the monitor and not always need to get out of bed.

When choosing a baby monitor, look for the following features:

- A visual light display as well as sound, which allows you to monitor your baby even with the volume turned down.

- Monitors work using radio channels, so choose a model with two channels, which allows you to switch channels if there is interference.

- A rechargeable model is more expensive initially, but the saving on batteries will make it cheaper in the long run.

- A low-battery indicator and an out-of-range indicator.

Baby sling

Some parents swear by this method of moving around with their babies. I never use one as I find it too big a strain on my back to carry a baby around like this for any length of time. Very small babies are also inclined to go straight to sleep the minute you hold them close to your chest, which defeats the whole purpose of my routines – i.e. keeping the baby awake at certain times of the day, and teaching the baby the right associations of going to sleep on his own. I do think that as babies get bigger, slings are a very useful way for parents to carry them around, especially when the baby is old enough to face forward.

If you feel a sling would be useful, here are some guidelines to observe when choosing one:

- The sling must have safety tabs to ensure it cannot come undone.

- It must provide your baby with enough head and neck support; some come with a detachable cushion that gives extra support for very young babies.

- It should offer the choice of baby facing inwards or outwards and have a seat with an adjustable height position.

- It should be made of strong, washable fabric with comfortable, padded shoulder straps.

- I would certainly recommend trying it on in the shop and putting a baby into it – one size does not fit all!

Baby chair

While many parents use the car seat in the house for their baby to sit in during the day, recent research has shown that newborn babies should not be put to sleep in the house in a car seat, as this can put them at risk of breathing difficulties (see page 12). So having an appropriate second seat for your baby in the early days is essential and it can also save you from having to move seats from room to room.

Baby seats come in different styles. Some chairs are rigid, with adjustable seat positions and a base that can either remain stable or be set to rocking mode. Another type is known as a 'bouncy chair'. This type is made of a lightweight frame covered in fabric and is designed to bounce as the baby moves. I have found them to be very popular with babies over two months, but they can make tiny babies feel insecure. Whatever type of chair you choose, make sure your baby is securely strapped in and never left unattended. Also, always place the baby on the floor when in a seat; never be tempted to leave him on a table or work-top, as the movement of the baby can easily shift the chair to the edge.

Here are some further guidelines:

- The frame and base should be firm and sturdy, and fitted with a strong safety strap.
- Choose one with an easily removable and washable cover.
- Buy a head support cushion for tiny babies.

Playpen

Playpens are frowned upon by some 'baby experts', who feel they hinder a baby's natural instinct to explore. My own feeling is that, while babies should never be left for long periods in a playpen, they can be very useful for ensuring your child is safe when you are preparing lunch or need to answer the door. If you do decide to use a playpen, I would recommend getting your baby used to it from a young age. A travel cot can be used as a playpen but, if you have the space, I would recommend the square wooden type, which is larger and would enable your baby to move around and pull himself up. Whichever sort you choose, make sure it is situated out of reach of hazards such as radiators, curtains and trailing flexes. Never hang toys on pieces of string or cord in the playpen, as these could prove fatal if your baby were to get tangled up.

Important points to look for when choosing a playpen:

- Check that there are no sharp metal hinges or catches on which your baby could harm himself.
- If choosing a mesh-type playpen or travel cot, make sure that the mesh is strong enough to prevent your baby from pushing small toys through and making a hole big enough to trap his hand or fingers.

Equipment needed for breast-feeding

Nursing bra

These are bras made with specially designed cups that can either be unhooked or unzipped to make breast-feeding easier. It is important that whatever style of bra you choose fits well. A good nursing bra should preferably be made of cotton for comfort, have wide, adjustable shoulder straps to help support your breasts and should not press tightly against the nipples, as this can be a cause of blocked milk ducts. I would suggest buying two before the birth. If they prove comfortable after your milk has come in, a further two can be purchased.

Breast pads

In the early days you will use a lot of breast pads, as they need to be changed every time your baby feeds. Many mothers prefer the round ones, contoured to fit the breasts. You may need to experiment with different brands, but sometimes the more expensive ones offer better absorbency, so can work out better value in the long run.

Nursing pillow

These pillows are shaped to fit around a mother's waist, bringing small babies up to the perfect height for breast-feeding. They can also be used for propping babies up and make an excellent back support for older babies who are learning to sit up. If you decide to invest in one, make sure it has a removable, machine-washable cover.

Nipple cream and sprays

These are designed to care for the breasts and help relieve any pain caused by breast-feeding. The main cause of pain, however, is poor positioning of the baby on the breast. If you experience pain either during or after feeding, it would be wise to consult your health visitor or breast-feeding counsellor for advice before purchasing a cream or spray. No other special creams or soaps are recommended when breast-feeding. Simply wash your breasts twice a day with plain water and after each feed. The nipples should be rubbed with a little breast milk and allowed to airdry.

Electric expressing machine

I am convinced that one of the reasons the majority of mothers I advise are successful at breast-feeding is because I encourage the use of an electric expressing machine. In the very early days when you are producing more milk than your baby may need (especially first thing in the morning), this can be expressed using one of these powerful machines. The expressed milk can then be stored in the fridge or freezer and used as a top-up later in the day when you are becoming tired and your milk supply may be low. This, I believe, is one of the main reasons why so many babies are restless and will not settle after their bath in the evening. If you want to breast-feed and quickly establish your baby in a routine, an electric breast pump will be a big asset. Do not be tempted by one of the smaller hand versions, which can be so inefficient as to put many women off expressing at all.

Freezer bags

Specially designed, pre-sterilised bags are an ideal way to store expressed breast milk and are available from chemists or baby departments in the larger stores and in large super markets. For details of how to store breast milk see guidelines on the NHS website: nhs.uk.

Feeding bottles

Most breast-feeding counsellors are against newborn babies being given a bottle, even of expressed milk. They claim that it creates nipple confusion, reducing the baby's desire to suck on the breast, leading in turn to poor milk supply and the mother giving up breast-feeding altogether. My own view is that the majority of women give up breast-feeding because they are totally exhausted with 'demand-feeding', often several times a night. I advise giving babies a bottle of either expressed milk or formula milk from the first week and introducing it by the fourth week at the latest. This one bottle can be given either last thing in the evening or during the night by someone other than the mother, thereby allowing the mother to sleep for several hours at a stretch. This, in turn, is likely to make her more able to cope with breast-feeding. I have never had a problem with a baby rejecting the mother's breast or becoming confused between nipple and teat, but this could happen if, in the early days, a baby was offered more than one bottle a day. Other good reasons for getting your baby used to a bottle are: firstly, it gives you some flexibility; secondly, the problem of later introducing bottles to an exclusively breast-fed baby doesn't arise; and thirdly, it gives the baby's father a wonderful opportunity to become more involved.

There are many types of bottle available, all claiming to be the best. From experience, I always recommend a wide-necked design as it makes cleaning and filling easier. It is also worth looking around for bottles that are free of Bisphenol A (BPA) as some scientists believe that this chemical, common in clear plastic feeding bottles, can leach into the milk.

I suggest that you start off by using a newborn teat, which will encourage your baby to work as hard drinking milk from a bottle as when breast-feeding. However, using a teat that is too slow for your baby can lead to problems such as wind, so take your baby's lead on this and move on to a faster-flowing teat as soon as he seems to struggle – this may be as early as three weeks but usually occurs around the eight-week mark. For advice on sterilising equipment, please refer to the next section.

Equipment needed for bottle-feeding

Feeding bottles

For the reasons already mentioned, I would strongly advise buying the wide-necked bottles described above. If your baby is likely to take all his milk from a bottle, it is important that the risk of developing colic or wind is kept to a minimum. When called upon to help a baby with colic, I often see an immediate improvement simply by switching to these wide-necked bottles. The teat is designed to be flexible and it allows the baby to suckle as he would at the breast. The wide-necked bottles, in time, can also be adapted to become feeding beakers with soft spouts and handles. If your baby is being exclusively bottle-fed, I would advise that you start off buying five 240ml (8oz) bottles and three 120ml (4oz) bottles.

Teats

Most feeding bottles come with a slow-flow teat designed to meet the needs of newborns. By eight weeks I have found that most babies feed better from a medium-flow teat and it is worthwhile stocking up on these extra teats from the beginning.

Bottle brush

Proper and thorough cleaning of your baby's bottles is of the utmost importance. Try to choose a brush with an extra-long plastic handle, which will allow more force to be put into cleaning the bottles.

Teat brush

Most mothers find that the easiest way to clean a teat is by using their forefinger. However, if you have extra-long nails, it may be worthwhile investing in one of these brushes, although they too can damage the hole of the teat, resulting in the need to replace the teats more frequently. Short nails are probably the answer!

Washing-up bowl

It is easier to organise and keep track of what is sterilised if all the dirty bottles are washed and sterilised at the same time. You will need somewhere to put the rinsed-out bottles and teats until they are ready to be sterilised, and a large stainless steel or plastic bowl can be used for this purpose, preferably with a lid.

Steriliser

Whether breast- or bottle-feeding, it is essential that all bottles and expressing equipment be sterilised properly. There are three main methods of sterilisation: boiling equipment for 10 minutes in a large pan; soaking equipment in a sterilising solution for two hours and rinsing with boiling water; or using an electric steam steriliser. From experience, the easiest, fastest and most effective method is the steam steriliser, and it is well worth making this investment. A word of caution – don't be tempted to purchase a microwave version. This type of unit not only holds fewer bottles, but it becomes a complete nuisance when you have to remove it to use the microwave for other purposes.

Kettle

Obviously it is essential for making up feeds, so your kettle should be efficient and of sufficient size. If, for personal reasons, you decide to formula-feed right from the beginning you will spend a lot of time in the first year making up feeds. (See pages 73–5 for recent guidelines on making up formula feeds.) You might, therefore, consider investing in an extra kettle. The water for the formula needs to be fresh, boiled just once and left to cool for no more than 30 minutes, so that it remains at a temperature of at least 70°C. If someone comes along to make a cup of tea while you are waiting for your water to cool, you'll have to start all over again. This can drive you crazy so an extra kettle just for the baby's water is often a wise investment. If you're expecting twins, it is essential.

Clothes for the newborn

The range of babywear available in the shops is both delightful and bewildering. While it can be fun choosing garments for your baby, I would urge you to approach this particular area with caution. Newborn babies grow at an alarming rate and will outgrow most of their first-size clothes by the first month, unless they were very small at birth. Although it is important to have enough clothes to allow for frequent changing, if you have too many, most will never get worn. You will need to renew your baby's wardrobe at least three times in the first year, and even if you stick to the cheaper ranges, it will still be a costly business. I would advise you to buy only the basics before your baby arrives. You may receive clothing as gifts when your baby arrives and you will have plenty of opportunity for clothes shopping during the first year.

When choosing clothes for the first month, don't be tempted by brightly coloured underwear or sleepwear. Newborn babies have a tendency to leak from both ends and it is impossible to remove stains by washing at anything less than 60°C. Brightly coloured garments will soon lose their appearance if frequently washed at this temperature, so stick to white, and leave the brighter colours for the outer garments.

In general, keep clothing simple during the first month. Dressing your baby in little white vests and white baby-grows in the early days makes washing so much easier when you can stick everything into the same load. If possible, invest in a tumble dryer: it is well worth the expense and means that you do not have to worry about ironing if you remove everything from the dryer the minute it is dry. Listed below are the basic items you will need for the first couple of months.

Vests	6–8	Socks	4–6 pairs
Nightdresses or sleepsuits	4–6	Hats	2
Day outfits	4–6	Mittens	2 pairs
Swaddling blankets	3	Cardigans	2–3
Snowsuit for a winter baby	1	Jacket	1

Vests

A newborn baby would normally wear a vest in both winter and summer, except in very hot weather. The best fabric next to a baby's skin is 100 per cent cotton, and if you want your beautiful layette to retain its appearance after numerous hot washes, stick to plain white, or white with a pale colour pattern. The best style of vest to buy is a 'body suit', which fastens under your baby's legs, has short sleeves and an envelope-style neckline for easy dressing.

Nightwear

The most common type of sleepwear is an all-in-one suit or baby-grow. They are snug and save time on laundry, but they can be awkward if you have to struggle to get your otherwise settled baby out of one to change his nappy. For this reason, some mothers prefer nightdresses. As with vests, 100 per cent cotton is best, and the simpler the design, the better. Avoid anything with ties at the neck, and if there are ties at the bottom, remove them as they could get caught around your baby's feet.

Day outfits

During the first couple of months, the easiest thing to dress your baby in will be baby-grows, which usually come in packs of two or three. If possible, try to buy pure cotton and choose a style that opens up either across the back or inside the legs, to ensure you don't need to undress your baby fully at nappy change. Dungaree-style clothes, without feet and with matching T-shirts, are also useful. They will last a bit longer as your baby grows, and the tops can be interchanged if your baby dribbles a lot. Choose styles in soft velour for very young babies, rather than stiff cotton or denim.

Cardigans

If your baby is born in the summer, you could probably get away with just two cardigans, ideally in cotton. With a winter baby, it would be best to have at least three cardigans, preferably wool. As long as your baby has cotton garments next to his skin, there should be no cause for irritation, and the simpler the design, the better.

Socks

Simple socks in cotton or wool are the most practical for new babies. Fancy styles with ribbons should be avoided, as should any type of shoe, however cute, as they could harm your baby's soft bones.

Hats

In the summer, it is important that you buy a cotton hat with a brim to protect your baby's head and face from the sun. Ideally, the brim should go right round the back of the neck. In spring and autumn, knitted cotton hats are adequate on cooler days. During the winter, or on very cold days, I would suggest a warm wool or fleece hat. Many of these are lined with cotton, but if not, a thin cotton hat can be worn underneath to protect sensitive skin.

Mittens

Small babies do not like to have their hands covered up, as they use them extensively to touch, feel and explore everything in close contact. If, however, your baby has sharp nails or tends to scratch, you could try the fine cotton mitts made for this purpose. In very cold weather use woollen or fleece mitts, but again, put cotton ones underneath if your baby has sensitive skin.

Swaddling blanket

I firmly believe that during the first few weeks all babies sleep better when swaddled. Whether you choose a blanket or shawl to swaddle, it should always be made of lightweight pure cotton that has a slight stretch to it. To avoid overheating, always swaddle your baby in a single layer, and when sleeping swaddled, reduce the number of blankets on the cot.

It is, however, important that by six weeks you start to get your baby used to being half-swaddled, under the arms. Cot death rates peak between two and four months and overheating is thought to be a major factor. Always check that you are not putting too many layers on and that the temperature of the room remains between 16–20°C, as recommended by The Lullaby Trust.

How to swaddle your baby

(a) Place baby on a square shawl and take one side up, level with the back of the head.

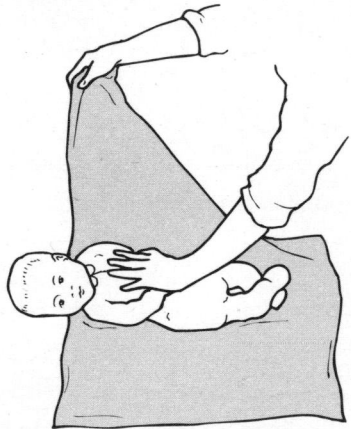

(b) Bring it down diagonally over the shoulder.

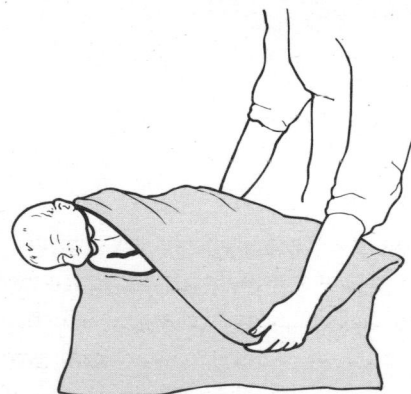

(c) Take the other side up, making it taut.

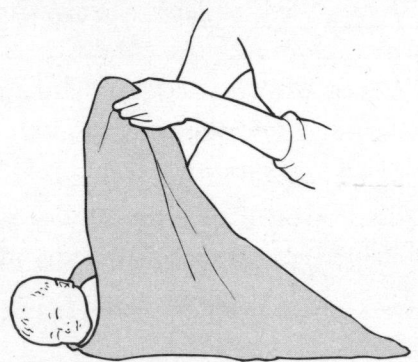

(d) Lift the baby a little and secure the end beneath his body.

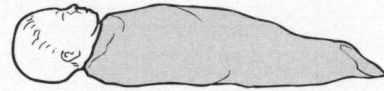

See www.contentedbaby.com for a video on how to swaddle correctly.

Snowsuit

When choosing snowsuits for your baby, always buy at least two sizes too big, as this allows plenty of room for growth. Avoid fancy designs with fur around the hood or dangling toggles, opting instead for one in an easy-care washable fabric. For tiny babies, poppers may be preferable to a zip, which can dig into the chin.

Jacket

A lightweight jacket can be useful for babies born at any time of the year. In summer it can be worn on chilly days, and in winter on milder ones. As with the snowsuits, choose one in a simple design in a washable fabric.

Your baby's laundry

Having spent a considerable amount of time and money on your baby's wardrobe, it is well worth the effort to be very fussy about caring for it. Because young babies grow out of their clothes so quickly, it should be possible, with good laundering, to pass them on to any brother or sister that follows. The following guidelines will help keep your baby's laundry in tip-top condition:

- Laundry should be sorted into different-coloured lots.

- Bedding, muslins and bibs need to be washed on a very hot wash to get rid of bacteria caused by milk stains and to eliminate the house dust mite, which can trigger allergies in very young babies.

- Load the washing machine no more than two-thirds full so that the clothes are rinsed thoroughly.

- Stains should always be treated before washing.

Whites: 60–90°C

Anything that is stained should be soaked overnight in a cold solution of Napisan, then washed at 60°C. Everything should be 100 per cent cotton, and bibs or towels with a coloured trim should have been tested for colour-run by washing separately for the first few washes. Sheets, muslins, vests, bibs, socks and white sleepsuits and nighties can also go in at 60°C if they are not very dirty. If they have not been soaked and are very dirty, they should go in a 90°C wash. Towels and face-cloths should be washed and dried together, and separate from other clothes, to avoid bobbling.

Light colours: 40°C

Most day clothes need only a very quick wash in the wool or delicate cycle. Anything stained should be soaked first overnight in cold water and Napisan, and rinsed before washing.

Dark colours: 30°C or handwash

Any dark outfits must be washed separately from the light colours even if they do not run; to mix the two will only result in the lighter colours taking on a grey tinge. Anything stained should be soaked first overnight in cold water and soap powder.

Woollens or delicates: handwash

Even if the label says 'machine wash', if the garment is very delicate or special, it is better to handwash using a very small amount of baby soap powder mixed with lukewarm water. Always squeeze the garment gently in the water when washing and rinsing; never wring, twist or allow a delicate garment to hang down. Rinse thoroughly in cold running water, gently squeeze out excess water, then roll in a clean, dry, white towel for a few hours. Finally, gently pull into shape and either dry flat or hang across a drying screen. Never hang up woollens from the bottom.

Use of the tumble dryer

Towels, bibs, fitted cot sheets and blankets can be tumble-dried, but flat cotton sheets should be dried so that they are slightly damp for easier and smoother ironing. Avoid drying towels and clothes together as it causes bobbling. Remove all clothes from the dryer and fold them as soon as possible to avoid creasing, and ensure that all clothes are properly aired.

Corduroy and dark clothes

To avoid fading and shadowing, dry these on the cool wash cycle for no more than 15 minutes. Then pull the clothes into shape and hang them up on hangers to dry. In this way they may not need to be ironed.

Ironing

Flat cot sheets and draw sheets should be ironed slightly damp for a smooth finish. Light-coloured outfits should be ironed using the water spray, and dark colours must be ironed on the inside with a very cool iron. Knitwear should be pressed with a muslin cloth. Ensure that all labels are ironed flat.

2

Why Follow a Routine?

t is nearly 19 years since I first typed the words, 'Why follow a routine?' Little did I know then the controversy those four simple words would create. But here I am, years later, explaining again why I think routine is important. I must stress that my views have not changed one little bit from when I wrote my first book. I personally believe that the majority of babies thrive and are happier in a routine. But I certainly realise and respect that following a routine is not a choice for all parents. There is already so much advice out there for 'baby-led parenting'; therefore, the advice I give in my books is for those parents who believe that they and their baby will be happier in a routine. I assume that one of the reasons you are reading this book is that you already have a certain level of structure in your life, and that you believe you will cope with your baby better by following some sort of routine. If this is the case then I can assure you that following Contented Little Baby routines will most certainly benefit both you and your baby. They are followed successfully by over a million parents around the world. Follow your own instinct as a parent as to what works best for you and your baby; use the routines and advice in this book as tools to help you be the parents that you want to be.

Why the CLB routines are different

During the years that I worked as a maternity nurse I read hundreds of books on child care, but I have also had the most unique privilege of working personally with more than 300 families around the world. It is because of these parents and their beautiful babies that I feel I am able to share with you so much of what I have learned, which I hope will help you overcome many of the everyday practicalities of parenting.

As a maternity nurse I would arrive at a home a few days after the birth, and live with the family 24/7 for periods of between 3–5 days, or sometimes several weeks to six months. While the media make much of the fact that many of my clients were rich and famous, I can assure you that the majority of families I helped were not. They often had to get outside help for health issues, family bereavement or other personal circumstances. Whether they lived in a mansion with 20 bedrooms or a flat with only one bedroom, were a rock or movie star, a struggling actor, high-profile banker or teacher, these parents all had one thing in common – they each wanted to ensure that their baby was happy and contented, and that they could somehow manage to meet all of their baby's needs as well as cope with the demanding lives that they led. The leading child care books at that time all endorsed baby-led parenting and claimed that it was impossible to put a small baby into a routine. The implication was that if parents were even to attempt to put their baby in a routine they could seriously damage the child's health.

In my first book I said that, having successfully spent many years teaching parents how to put their newborns into a routine that results in a happy, thriving, contented baby, I can only assume that the authors of these books have not personally worked with enough babies to know this is possible. The fact that *The Contented Little Baby Book* became a runaway bestseller through personal recommendation is proof enough that the statement I made in my first edition in 1999 has been proved true. Parents who have properly read the book, the routines and the advice I give, can testify that the CLB routines do really work. Unlike old-fashioned four-hourly feeding they do not involve leaving a baby to yell until a feed is due, or leaving him to cry himself to sleep for lengthy periods. While establishing a routine is often very hard work and requires a lot of sacrifices on the part of the parents, millions of parents around the world will testify that it is worth it because they quickly learn how to meet the needs of their babies so that any distress is kept to a minimum.

Benefits for your baby

The reason that the CLB routines are different from traditional four-hourly routines is that they are created to meet the natural sleep and feeding needs of all healthy normal babies. They also allow for the fact that some babies need more sleep than others, and that some may be able to go longer between feeds than others. The aim of the routines is not to push your baby through the night without a feed, but to ensure that by structuring the feeding and sleeping during the day, your baby's night-time waking will be kept to a minimum. He will wake and feed quickly before settling back to sleep. The routines also ensure that once your baby is capable of going one longer spell between feeds, this will happen in the middle of the night, not during the day. The basis of these routines evolved over many years of observing babies in my care. Some babies would develop a feeding pattern very quickly with little prompting, while others would be difficult to feed and settle for many weeks. The main observations that I made from babies who settled quickly into a pattern were:

- The parents had a positive approach, wanted a routine, and tried to keep the first couple of weeks as calm as possible.

- Handling of the baby by visitors was kept to a minimum so that the baby felt relaxed and secure in his new surroundings (especially important when the baby is first brought home from hospital).

- The baby always had regular sleep times in a quiet room.

- The baby was kept awake for a short spell after the daytime feeds.

- When he was awake, and had been well fed and winded, he was then stimulated and played with for short periods.

- A bedtime routine was established from day one. He would be bathed at the same time every evening, then fed and settled in a quiet room. If the baby did not settle, the parents would ensure that they kept things as quiet as possible and continued to comfort him in a dimly lit room until he did eventually settle.

Benefits for you

One of the most stressful things any parent has to endure is to listen to their baby crying, particularly if the crying goes on for any length of time and all attempts to calm the baby fail. By following the CLB routines you will soon learn the signs of hunger, tiredness, boredom or indeed many of the other reasons that cause young babies to get upset. The fact that you are able to understand his needs and meet them quickly and confidently will leave both you and your baby calm and reassured, and avoid unnecessary crying. The common situation of fretful baby and fraught parents is avoided. The other big plus for parents following my routines is that they have free time in the evening to relax and enjoy each other's company. This is not usually possible for parents who follow baby-led parenting, as any attachment parenting website will show the early evening is a time when these babies are often particularly fretful and can require endless rocking and patting to try to keep them calm.

Other approaches

The routines and advice in this book evolved over many years. During my time as a maternity nurse I tried and tested various ways of establishing breast-feeding and healthy sleep habits. Before I further expand on why I believe that my methods are so successful, I will briefly discuss the other methods I have had experience with over the years, which I hope will give you an insight into why I believe that the CLB routines can be of great benefit to many parents and their babies.

Strict four-hourly feeding routine

This routine evolved when hospital birth took over from home birth several decades ago and women would stay in the maternity unit for up to 14 days. Their babies were brought to them from the nursery every four hours and given a strict 10–15 minutes on each breast before being returned to the nursery. Although such routines are more associated with our grand-mothers' generation, there are still parents nowadays who believe that babies can be slotted into them. During my early years of working as a maternity nurse I did work with some families that adopted these routines, and for some they did succeed, particularly if they were formula-fed.

However, I did find that trying to establish breast with a strict four-hourly feeding schedule, where feeds were limited to a 10–15 minutes on each breast, did not work for the majority of babies. The mother, believing that the reason her baby was not managing to stick to the schedule was because she was not producing enough milk, would very early be pressured to introduce top-up feeds of formula in order to get the baby to feed at the right times according to the routines. I would be a multimillionaire if I had a pound for every granny who has said to me, 'My milk dried up the minute I left the hospital.' The reality was that, due to rigid routines and restricted timing of feeds, the mother's milk had started to dry up long before she left the hospital. The trend for bottle-feeding became well established in the 1950s and 1960s, with many mothers not even attempting to breast-feed. This trend continued well into the 1970s. Then, as research started to unearth more and more information regarding the health benefits of breast-feeding, the trend started to swing back again. Mothers were told not to restrict feeds and to allow their babies to feed for as long as was needed to satisfy the baby's hunger. It is important that you understand the CLB routines are not about strict four-hourly feeding schedules. It could be many weeks before a four-hourly feeding pattern can emerge, and I would urge you not to be pressured into it, however keen you are to establish a routine. The main reasons four-hourly feeding can fail are:

- Six feeds a day in the early days are usually not enough to stimulate a good milk supply.

- Babies need to feed little and often in the early days; restricting feeding to six feeds may lead to your baby being short of his daily intake.

- Babies between one week and six weeks old usually need at least 30 minutes to reach the hind milk.

- Hind milk is at least three times higher in fat content than fore milk, and is essential for satisfying your baby's hunger.

Demand-feeding

Although I did look after some babies that were put into a strict four-hourly feeding routine from birth, much of my experience in the early days of my career was with babies who were being fed on demand.

The advice given then is the same nowadays. Mothers are encouraged to let their babies take the lead, allowing their babies to feed as often and for as long as they want. This method, like the four-hourly method of feeding, did succeed for some babies, but for a huge number that I was asked to help it did not work. One thing that became obvious very early in my experience is that, quite simply, many newborn babies do not demand to be fed. This is particularly true of low-birth-weight babies and twins. That is my main objection to demand-feeding. If you had had the experience of sitting by the bedside of a baby only days old fighting for his life because he has become seriously dehydrated through not being fed enough, you would probably feel the same way. Dehydration is a very serious problem among newborn babies and one that many new parents are now aware of. The production of breast milk works on a supply and demand basis, so babies who are allowed to sleep for long periods between feeds are not put to the breast often enough in a 24-hour period to signal the breasts to make enough milk. Mothers are lulled into a false sense of security that they have a baby who is easy and sleeps well.

In fact, what they have is a very sleepy baby who normally, 2–3 weeks down the line, will start waking up more often and demanding more milk than the mother is producing. A pattern quickly emerges of the baby having to feed every couple of hours, day and night, in order to have his daily nutritional needs met. The current advice is that this pattern is normal and that the baby will sort itself out, but mothers are not told that with some babies it may take months! Sometimes a pattern does occur where the baby will go longer between feeds. But this is often one where the baby is feeding so much in the night that when he does wake up for feeds during the day, they tend to be short, small feeds. This leads to a vicious circle of the baby needing to feed more in the night to satisfy his daily needs. The mother then becomes exhausted from several night-time wakings and not managing to rest enough during the day. This exhaustion can often lead to some or all of the following problems:

- Exhaustion and stress reduce the mother's milk supply, increasing the baby's need to feed little and often.

- Babies who continue to need to feed 10–12 times a day after the first week often become so exhausted from lack of quality sleep that they become even more tired, and feed for shorter and shorter periods at each feed.

- Exhaustion can lead to the mother being too tired to concentrate properly on positioning the baby correctly on the breast for any length of time.

- Poor positioning on the breast is the main reason for painful, and often cracked and bleeding nipples, which again reduces how well the baby feeds at the breast.

- A sleepy baby left too long between feeds in the early days reduces the mother's chances of being able to building up a good milk supply.

Another reason I am so opposed to the term 'demand-feeding' is that it is often taken too literally. Every time the baby cries it is fed and mothers are not taught to look for other reasons why the baby may be crying – overstimulation or overtiredness, for example. Of course, all babies must be fed if they are hungry; no baby should be left to cry for a feed or kept to a strict timetable if he is genuinely hungry. But in my experience, and if research on sleeping problems in this country is anything to go by, a huge number of demand-fed babies do not automatically fall into a healthy sleeping pattern months down the line. Many continue to wake up and feed little and often, long after a time when they are capable of going a longer spell in the night. Another problem is that babies who continue to feed little and often invariably end up being fed to sleep. This creates a whole other set of sleeping problems, where they have learned the wrong sleep associations and cannot get to sleep without being fed.

Whether you are the parent of a newborn baby or an older baby I would urge you not even to attempt to start the routines until you have read and understood Chapters 3 and 4 on feeding and sleeping in the first year. Because CLB routines are not like the old-fashioned four-hourly routines, it is not just a case of reading a routine and trying to fit your baby's feeding and sleeping into the times I suggest. The CLB routines change 10 times during the first year. The times given for feeding and sleeping in each set of the routines are approximate guidelines for your baby's age, not rigid rules. You need to understand the principles behind the routines so that you can make slight adjustments to ensure that your baby's individual needs are being met.

Your questions answered

Q I am six months pregnant and, like many new mothers-to-be, I am concerned about how I am going to cope with the sleepless nights. My antenatal class stresses the importance of demand-feeding, that new babies should be fed when they need it and that I should not attempt a routine in the early days. I am concerned that if I try to follow your routines, I may be denying my baby food when he is really hungry.

A The CLB routines are not about denying babies a feed when they are really hungry. Quite the opposite. My main concern about demand-feeding with very young babies is that a great many babies do not demand to be fed in the very early days. This can lead to many serious problems, the main one being that a baby who is not feeding from the breast will not stimulate the breast to produce enough milk. We therefore arrive at the situation, three or four weeks down the line, where a mother is trying to feed her baby and not producing enough milk. A vicious circle then evolves where the mother is feeding the baby every 1–2 hours, night and day, to try to satisfy his needs – but by this time, exhaustion has set in. This is one of the main reasons why the milk supply decreases and women find they have to stop breast-feeding. In the very early days I always advise a mother to assume that, if the baby is crying, then hunger is possibly the main reason why, and the baby should be fed. However, I do stress that if a baby is continually crying and unhappy, then you should also look for reasons why the baby cannot last the three hours between feeds. Often the baby has not been latched on properly to the breast and, while he may appear to be constantly sucking for up to an hour, much

> **Top Tip**
>
> Always remember that three-hourly feeding means you count three hours from the beginning of one feed to the beginning of the next, irrespective of how long the feed itself takes.

of the time he is not actually drinking well. This is why mothers who are breast-feeding and finding that their baby is not going happily for 2–3 hours between feeds should always seek advice from an experienced breast-feeding counsellor. The majority of healthy babies weighing more than 2.7kg (6lbs) at birth, who regain their birth weight within a couple of weeks and are putting on around 180g a week, should manage to go three hours (or perhaps a little more) between feeds but this will only happen if the baby receives enough milk to satisfy his needs.

Q Do I really have to wake my newborn baby up to feed him? He wants to sleep all the time and I am tempted to leave him.

A I do understand. It is a great temptation when you are tired from the birth to catch up on rest during the daytimes while your baby sleeps. But your baby will only be this sleepy for a few short weeks and he will then increasingly want to be awake, playing and having social time with you and others. He won't know the difference between day and night, and unless you gently guide him into a routine, you could end up with him wide awake and wanting to play games at 4am. So, yes, I do stress the importance of implementing three-hourly feeding (or sooner if your baby is hungry) during the first week to ensure that the breasts are stimulated enough to increase the mother's milk production. Waking the baby three-hourly throughout the day will ensure that the baby will more than likely only wake once in the night between 12am and 6am. A mother who is well-rested and relaxed will be much more likely to produce a more abundant milk supply than a mother who is tired and stressed. In the long term you will both benefit from establishing this pattern.

Q Several friends and relations have said that it is cruel to wake a sleeping baby and that he will wake up when he is ready to feed. I am a very organised person and feel that following a routine would be best for both my baby and me, but I am frightened that I could do some sort of psychological or physical damage to my baby by waking him.

A It is obvious that the people who say it is cruel to wake a sleeping baby to feed him have never had to care for very premature or sick babies as I have. Waking these babies on a regular basis so they fed little and often was the only way to ensure their survival. Over the years, watching these babies grow up into young children, I have never seen any of them showing any psychological or physical damage. I am convinced that there is a bigger risk of such damage to both baby and mother if a situation arises where a baby is up and demanding to be fed every hour in the night. In the early days I advise feeding a baby little and often to establish breast-feeding. Sometimes this will involve waking him but I advise that, should a young baby demand feeding before three hours, then he must, of course, be fed. A pattern will quickly be established for both you and your baby from which you will both benefit.

Q The current advice is that parents should have their baby in the same room as them for all sleeps, for the first six months. I am concerned that my baby will not sleep well in our living room for naps and in the evening and that it will be difficult to get him used to sleeping in his nursery when he does reach six months. How easy is it to establish your routines while also adhering to the new guidelines?

A The latest advice is that your baby should be put down for all his sleeps in the room you are in until he is six months old during the day and at night. However, getting your baby used to his own room sooner rather than later can help you avoid disrupting and unsettling him when he reaches six months. You can make the nursery a peaceful haven for him by using it for nappy changing, feeding and wind-down or quiet play time.

In terms of settling your baby to sleep in your living space, try to keep things as quiet as possible for him to help distinguish between 'awake' time and time for sleeping. Keep everything calm and quiet. It is unlikely that you will have a cot both in your bedroom and in your living space, therefore a pram with a proper firm mattress would be an acceptable option. Follow the same guidelines for settling your baby in the pram as those given for settling him in a cot: place him in the pram with his feet at the bottom, and firmly tuck in any sheets and blankets. Putting the hood up during sleep times will help keep out the light and help your baby to sleep better.

Lastly, remember that these recommendations are only for the first six months, and that after that time you can start to settle your baby in his own room for naps and night-time sleep (see page 240 for advice on how to make the transition easier for him).

Q Is it true that you say that babies should not be cuddled? I keep reading that babies need lots of physical affection and attention in order for them to feel secure.

A I have always stressed the importance of physical contact and affection with your baby. However, I do say that parents should make sure that the cuddling and affection they give is to satisfy their baby's emotional needs before their own. Sometimes when a baby is crying, it is because he just needs to go to sleep; too much cuddling when he is tired can simply make your baby more tired and irritable. And, crucially, there is a difference between cuddling your baby and cuddling him to sleep. If he gets used to the latter, it will create a dependence that you will have to break at some point – and it is much easier to get him used to settling himself to sleep at three weeks of age than three months or three years.

Q While I would like a routine when my baby is born, I do not want to leave him to cry for long spells.

A I would never advise that young babies should be left to cry for lengthy periods of time to get themselves to sleep. I do stress that some overtired babies will fight sleep and they should be allowed 5–10 minutes' 'crying-down' period. They should *never* be left for any longer than this before they are checked again. I also stress that a baby should never be left crying for even 2–3 minutes if there is any doubt that he could be hungry or need winding. With some babies who have reached six months or a year and are waking several times a night because they have learned the wrong sleep associations, brought on by demand-feeding or being rocked or cuddled to sleep, it may be that some form of sleep training needs to be used.

In my book, *Your Baby and Toddler Problems Solved*, I stress that any form of sleep training is always a last resort to get a baby over six months to sleep during the night and should only ever be used once parents are absolutely sure that the baby is not waking up because he is hungry, or he is sleeping too much during the day. The majority of sleep problems that I deal with through my consultancy are nearly always resolved without controlled crying because, by ensuring that parents get the feeding and sleeping right, in the majority of cases the baby will start to sleep better and longer naturally at night. However, if a baby has learned the wrong sleep associations and has to be constantly rocked or fed to sleep, then sometimes the only solution is some form of sleep training. It is important that before commencing sleep training you take your baby to see the GP to check there are no medical problems. The whole aim of the CLB routines is to ensure from the very beginning that the baby's needs are being met so that he does not need to cry for any length of time. The guidelines I give are also to help mothers understand the different reasons why a baby may cry. If a baby is in a routine from a very early age the mother will quickly learn to understand and hence anticipate his needs. I have found that this results in the baby crying very seldom – around 5–10 minutes a day in my experience, and only for a very short period until they have learned to self-settle themselves.

Q I have read that on your routines a baby should not be fed in the middle of the night once he reaches 12 weeks. Surely all babies are different and a baby should not be forced to go without food if he is really hungry?

A Some babies, particularly breast-fed babies, may need to be fed around 5/6am until they are fully weaned, which can be anywhere up to seven or eight months of age. The majority of babies I have cared for personally would sleep through the night (i.e. from the late feed to 6–7am) somewhere between eight and twelve weeks. The huge feedback that I receive from readers would indicate that this does seem to be the average age at which babies forming routines would sleep for a longer spell. Each baby, of course, is an individual, but if your baby does not sleep through the night until he is seven months old, neither you, nor I, nor your baby has 'failed'. My routines are there to help you begin to structure your days and nights, and perseverance will pay off when your baby is ready. How quickly a baby sleeps through the night is very much determined by his weight and the amount of milk he is capable of drinking at each feed during the day. Some babies who are only capable of drinking small amounts at each feed would obviously need a feed in the night for longer than a baby who is capable of drinking a larger amount at each feed during the day. The aim of the CLB routines is not to push the baby through the night as quickly as possible or to deny the baby a feed in the night if he genuinely needs it. It is to ensure that the baby receives most of his nutritional needs during the day so that when he is physically and mentally ready to go through the night he will automatically do so. The feedback I have had, along with my many years of experience caring for babies, confirms this approach works.

Q I read a message from a mother in an Internet parenting chatroom that she is very lonely and depressed following your routines as it leaves her no time to get out and meet other mothers.

A I have always said that putting a young baby into a routine can be very demanding on the parents, particularly in the early weeks. However, by the time a baby is 2–3 months of age, a pattern has usually emerged where the baby can stay awake for longer periods during the day and sleep for longer periods at night. In my experience of working with thousands of mothers, their social outings were certainly restricted for the first 2–3 weeks but after that I cannot recall many mothers who did not manage to meet their friends most afternoons between 2pm and 5pm or at playgroups in the mornings. It is important not just to read the routine for your baby's age, but also the whole concept of the routines as found in the feeding and sleeping chapters (3 and 4 respectively). Once you have an understanding of how the routines work, you will then find that you are able to tweak and adjust routines during the day, without it affecting the night-time sleep. The mothers I have worked with have all felt that it is worth putting in the hard work at the beginning because the result is a contented baby who sleeps well at night and enjoys his social times during the day. A mother who has had a good night's sleep will be able to enjoy her days more, too!

I always advise mothers, in the early days, to try to ensure that at least every second day they arrange for a friend or relative to come and visit them so that they do not feel lonely or abandoned. I also stress the importance of a walk every day with the baby to get some fresh air. You can do this with friends – and chatting in the park is also a great way to meet other parents.

Q **In your routines you tell mothers when to eat and drink. This strictness puts me off.**

A From my experience; in the early days mothers are often exhausted and put their own needs – even the basics like eating and drinking – at the bottom of their list of priorities. Struggling with a newborn on your own can mean that you find yourself at teatime having only had a piece of toast and half a cup of tea. As a nursing mum, you need to eat plenty of food regularly and to drink plenty of water in order to produce enough milk for your baby and to keep up your own energy levels. I know that many people using my routines refer to the book several times a day so the hours suggested for breakfast, lunch and for drinking lots of water are just a gentle reminder not to neglect yourself – and they fit in with what your baby is doing, helping make it easier for you to care for yourself, too.

Q Why are your routines so rigid? Surely half an hour here or there won't make much difference?

A *The New Contented Little Baby Book* contains over 10 different routines taking you from week one of your baby's life, right up to the end of his first year. They have been carefully compiled to allow for the fact that your baby will be growing and changing. As he goes through his first three months, he will gradually need less and less daytime sleep as he will be enjoying being awake and sociable. He needs stimulation and fun during the day. He will need weaning at some point (current guidelines recommend exclusive breast-feeding for six months). His sleeping and feeding needs are constantly changing throughout his first year of life. In my experience, adapting to your baby's changing needs is best done slowly and steadily. My routines are specific in order to help you to make those gradual changes. Once your baby is sleeping for 12 hours every night, you will feel a huge sense of relief and he will be getting the long, deep sleep that he needs for healthy growth and development. My routines are designed around babies' natural rhythms and they work. You do not have to stick rigidly to them, but half an hour can have a knock-on effect which disrupts the rest of your day and, possibly, your night. For example, if your day begins nearer 8am than 7am, you will find your baby has a later nap at around 1pm. If he doesn't wake until after 3pm you will find it difficult to get him to settle at 7pm, as he is unlikely to be sleepy by then. If the last feed of the day is nearer 8pm, you could find as a result that he does not want his 10pm feed and will wake up in the night. This is certainly not the end of the world occasionally but, over a period of time and as his nutritional needs change, you could find night waking continues, leaving you exhausted and less able to enjoy your baby.

Q I have been trying to follow your routines for four weeks but my baby is not remotely near fitting in with them. I feel like a failure and wonder if I should just give up and let her feed and sleep whenever she wants.

A It can be very difficult in the early days, and many parents understandably feel it would be easier on them if they let the baby decide what she wants to do. Bear in mind you are recovering from the birth, and looking after a baby, routine or not, is extremely hard work. My routines make sure the hard work is limited to as short a period as possible. Think how hard it would be if your baby was still waking up in the night at nine months old. I can assure you it is worth persevering.

Don't necessarily expect instant contentment, but the result of sticking with the routines in the first weeks is a more enjoyable babyhood and toddlerhood for you and your child. When your baby does fit in, and she will very soon, I can guarantee you will never regret the effort you put in to follow the routines in the first few weeks. The routines are there to help guide you and your baby into what represents the baby's natural patterns and rhythms. Remember that you are not 'failing' if your baby doesn't fit in; just keep going, taking a day at a time. As every experienced parent and grandparent will be telling you – the first few months go very quickly.

Start each day at 7am and attempt to follow the day's routine, but if it has gone pear-shaped by lunchtime, because your baby is wide awake at nap time and sleepy during the social times I suggest, don't panic. Keep repeating the same pattern of feeds and sleeps every day as best you can and your baby will pick it up very soon. If she is crying for food before the recommended time and you have tried distracting her or playing with her then you must, of course, feed her. If you really cannot rouse her from a sleep when it's time to play, don't give yourself or her a hard time. I found that by getting the baby up out of the cot when they are meant to be awake and having them in a bright room on their play mat, they will eventually wake up naturally, which is better than trying to force them to wake up. Looking after a baby on your own without the support of family close at hand can be very hard work. You are not alone in going through the experience, however, and you are certainly not a failure – it will get better!

Q Why are you so strict about avoiding eye contact at the late feed? I feel very cruel depriving my baby of cuddles and this close contact.

A Please don't deprive your baby of cuddles! Nowhere do I suggest you should not cuddle your baby. On the contrary, a baby who is being held close to his mother, whether breast-fed or bottle-fed, will enjoy his feed more and be ready to return to a contented sleep after he has been winded and settled down quietly. I advise avoiding too much eye contact, especially near the end of this feed, to ensure that he settles quickly. Your cuddles can be very close, but overstimulating him at wind-down time can cause him to become overtired and not settle well. He needs his sleep for his mental and physical development and without it he could become fretful, irritable and inconsolable. I feel it is better for the baby to be played with, sung to, shown interesting toys and books when he is wide awake during the day. Cuddling must be about your baby's needs and not just your own.

Q Your routines are so strict. When can I enjoy my baby without worrying about what he should be doing next?

A I sincerely hope that every parent enjoys his or her baby, from the first exciting day they come home from hospital, right through babyhood, toddlerhood and beyond. Every day is filled with opportunities for cuddling, playing, singing, reading, splashing in the bath, tickling toes while nappy changing and chatting to your baby. But it is beyond doubt that a contented baby who is well-fed and rested at the right times is best able to appreciate and participate in these activities. My routines are there to support and help you find a structure to your days that will result in a contented baby, and once you get to understand them better you will see that they are not really so strict. Having a routine allows you the opportunity to have a much better social life than if you don't know from one day to the next when your baby is going to feed or sleep. I appreciate and respect that routines are not for everyone, however, and if you feel stressed by following a routine then stop trying for a few days and then see how you feel having less structure in your day. The aim of my routines is to help you have a contented, happy baby and also to help you avoid long-term problems such as: overtiredness due to over-stimulation; sleep association where a baby has to be rocked to sleep or driven round the block; or continual night wakings which leave you feeling exhausted each morning. Should any of these problems develop, you could turn to my book later on for help.

Bonding evolves slowly over many weeks, and for many mothers without help or support there can be, along with feelings of joy and love for a new baby, feelings of sheer exhaustion, failure and frustration. Nights of broken sleep do not help and mothers often contact me because they feel guilty and resentful that they are not enjoying their babies. Weeks of sleep-deprivation caused by endless middle-of-the-night feeding is bound to hamper bonding and enjoyment of your baby. My routines are there to help you and your baby, not to cause stress, anxiety or feelings of inadequacy. Understanding them will help enormously.

Q I have a toddler as well as a new baby to care for and I cannot seem to get your routines to work around both of them.

A This is an important point and I have covered adapting routines to fit in with school runs and older children in my books *The Contented Toddler Years* and *The Contented Baby with Toddler Book*. Many mothers find that school runs or nursery for older children mean that the nap times I suggest are not workable. If you used my routines with your first child, you will at least find the 7am start and 7pm bedtime already established in your household. Your toddler may still take a lunchtime nap if he is under three and this can combine nicely with the baby's nap. You might even get an overlap of half an hour to yourself! I suggest that you concentrate on sticking to my suggested total amounts of daytime sleep. So if you have to adapt your baby's daytime sleep around your toddler's routine, try not to let the baby exceed the recommended amount of daily sleep. Then bedtime will at least be guaranteed and you can have an evening to rest and recover from caring for two young children.

3

Milk Feeding in the First Year

Milk feeding is of vital importance during the first year of your baby's life. It not only helps lay the foundation for your baby's future health, but it also plays a huge part in how well your child sleeps. I hope that the advice in this book will help you successfully establish breast-feeding for your baby, and even if it does not appeal to you, that you will at least give it a try. Many mothers I have helped who were totally stressed when breast-feeding their first baby because of the exhaustion of demand feeding, found breast-feeding their second a complete pleasure when following my CLB routines. If, for some reason, you have already given up or have chosen not to breast-feed, I still offer lots of advice on how to get bottle-feeding right. The whole aim of my book, and the advice within, is to help and support parents, and in particular mothers, who I know feel a huge amount of pressure these days about giving their baby the best start in life. Of course, breast milk is best, but the reality is that if formula were not a good substitute it would have been banned by the health authorities years ago. So if you have already given up breast-feeding or made a personal informed choice not to, please do not be made to feel guilty by the opinions of others who disapprove. Ignore any nasty comments that you will not bond so closely with your baby because you are not breast-feeding. Speaking from personal experience, my own mother only managed to breast-feed me for about 10 days, and no mother and daughter could have been closer than we were. Equally, I have friends who were breast-fed for nearly two years and cannot stand the sight of their mothers!

However, I must stress that, contrary to advice from well-meaning relations, bottle-feeding does not necessarily guarantee you a more contented baby, or make it easier to put him into a routine. Whether your baby is breast-fed or bottle-fed, it will still take time and perseverance to establish a routine, so please do not choose or change your baby's feeding to formula, thinking that you will have a more contented baby. A bottle-fed baby will need as much guidance and help into a routine as a breast-fed one, the only difference being that all the responsibility normally lies with the mother who is breast-feeding. For mothers who wish to breast-feed, the CLB routines will allow you to breast-feed successfully and have a routine, with the bonus of your partner being able to give your baby a bottle of expressed milk.

Why breast-feeding goes wrong

The first thing that became obvious to me very early on when working with new mothers is that, while breast-feeding may be the most natural way to feed a newborn baby, for all mothers it does not come easily. Immediately after the birth, midwives encourage mothers to put their baby straight to the breast, and guide them through the techniques of positioning and latching the baby on. For some mothers their baby will latch on to the breast easily, feed well and then drop off to sleep easily until the next feed. For others the baby will fuss and fret, fight the breast or take several sucks before falling asleep. These problems are all very common in the early days. Mothers are now discharged from hospital within 48 hours of giving birth, and many are sent home without having grasped the basic latching-on techniques that are essential if breast-feeding is to be a success. When I worked as a maternity nurse I would often arrive at a family's home to find a mother with nipples that were so cracked and bleeding that she would be in tears every time she put the baby to her breast. In situations like this, breast-feeding and bonding get off to a very bad start for both mother and baby. The mother is in a lot of physical pain and also suffers mental agony, thinking she is not a good enough mother because her baby is not latching on properly. The baby gets stressed and cries a lot through hunger, because he is not feeding well enough. All of these problems, and many others associated with breast-feeding, could be avoided if more attention and help were given to the mother in the early days.

I am alarmed by some of the advice being given to new mothers in this country today regarding feeding their newborns. They are told within hours of giving birth that they should use their natural instinct and that their baby will let them know what he needs. I have been fortunate enough to have worked with many families in the Far East and Middle East, where they sometimes seem to know more about what really matters in the early days after the birth, i.e. that both mother and baby need as much help and support as possible. The attitude of families from these countries is often totally different from the one we adopt in this country. The mother and baby spend the early days getting as much rest and sleep as possible, and mothers eat a special diet to ensure that they are eating enough of the right foods to help produce a good milk supply. Babies are not just thrust upon their mothers' breasts then left, because 'mother and baby will both do what comes naturally'. Whether it was from a professional outside source as well as myself, or members of the extended family, the mothers with whom I worked usually had someone to help them with the latching on and feeding position in the early days.

I believe passionately that the way to ensuring more mothers breast-feed successfully is to give them help in the early days. While breast-feeding does come naturally to many mothers, it does not come naturally to all, and we need to take this into account when we give advice.

How milk is produced and the composition of breast milk will also help you understand how the CLB feeding routines can and will work with breast-feeding, provided that you follow the advice on adjusting the routines to meet increased demand during growth spurts, or at times when your baby has not taken a full feed. The following brief summary gives an overview of how breast milk is produced. For more in-depth information I would recommend that you read *What to Expect When You're Breast-Feeding ... And What If You Can't?* by Clare Byam-Cook.

Milk production

Milk let-down reflex

The hormones produced during your pregnancy help prepare your breasts for the production of milk. Once your baby is born and put to the breast to suck, a hormone called oxytocin is released from the pituitary gland at the base of your brain, which sends a 'let-down' signal to the breast. The muscles supporting the milk glands contract and the milk is pushed down the 15 or 20 milk ducts as the baby sucks. Many women feel a slight tingling in their breasts, and their womb contracting when their milk lets down. These feelings normally disappear within a week or two. You may also experience a let-down when you hear your baby cry, or if you think about him when you are apart. If you get tense or are very stressed, oxytocin is not released, making it difficult for your milk to let down. Therefore, it is essential for successful breast-feeding that you feel calm and relaxed. This can be helped by preparing everything needed for a feed in advance. Make sure you are sitting comfortably with your back straight, and that the baby is well-supported. Take time to position him on to the breast correctly. Pain caused by incorrect positioning also affects oxytocin being released, which in turn affects the let-down reflex.

Milk composition

The first milk your breasts will produce is called colostrum. It is higher in protein and vitamins and lower in carbohydrate and fat than the mature milk that comes in between the third and fifth day. Colostrum also contains some of your antibodies, which will help your baby resist any infections you have had. Compared to the mature milk that soon follows, colostrum is much thicker and looks more yellow. By the second to third day, the breasts are producing a mixture of colostrum and mature milk. Then, somewhere between the third and fifth day, the breasts become engorged, and they will feel very hard, tender and often painful to the touch. This is a sign that the mature milk is fully in. The pain is caused not only by the milk coming in, but also by the enlargement of the milk glands in the breasts and the increased blood supply to the breasts. When the milk comes in, it is essential to feed your baby little and often. Not only will it help stimulate a good milk supply, but it will also help relieve the pain of engorgement. During this time it may be difficult for your baby to latch on to the breast and it may be necessary to express a little milk before feeding. This can be done by placing warm, wet flannels on the breasts and gently expressing a little milk by hand. Many mothers also find some relief by placing the leaves of a chilled cabbage inside their bras between feeds.

Mature milk looks very different from colostrum. It is thinner and looks slightly blue in colour, and its composition also changes during the feed. At the beginning of the feed, your baby gets the fore milk, which is high in volume and low in fat. As the feed progresses, your baby's sucking will slow down and he will pause for longer between sucks. This is a sign that he is reaching the hind milk. Although he only gets a small amount of hind milk, it is very important that he is left on the breast long enough to reach it. It is this hind milk that will help your baby go longer between feeds. If you transfer him to the second breast before he has totally emptied the first breast, he will be more likely to get two lots of fore milk. This will have a knock-on effect and leave him feeling hungry again in a couple of hours. Another feed of fore milk will quickly lead to your baby becoming very 'colicky'. While some babies do not get enough from only one breast and need to be put on the second breast, always check that he has completely emptied the first breast before transferring him (see page 62). I find that at the end of the first week, by making sure babies are given around 25 minutes on the first breast, and offered the second breast for 5–15 minutes, I can be sure that they are getting the right balance of fore milk and hind milk. It also ensures that they are content to go between 3–4 hours before demanding their next feed. If your baby is feeding from both breasts at each feed, always remember to start the next feed on the breast you last fed from, so that you can be certain each breast is totally emptied every second feed.

In order to encourage a quick and easy let-down, and to ensure that your baby gets the right balance of fore milk and hind milk, the following guidelines should help:

- Make sure that you rest as much as possible between feeds, and that you do not go too long between meals. Also, eat small, healthy snacks between meals.

- Prepare in advance everything needed for the feed: a comfortable chair with arms and a straight back, and perhaps a footstool. Cushions to support both you and the baby, a drink of water and some soothing music will all help towards a relaxing, enjoyable feed for both of you.

- It is essential that you take your time to position the baby on the breast correctly; poor positioning leads to painful and often cracked, bleeding nipples. This, in turn, can affect your let-down and result in a poor feed.

- Once the milk is in and you have built up the time your baby feeds from the breast, it is important that he is on the breast long enough to reach the hind milk. Some babies need up to 30 minutes to empty the breast. By gently squeezing your nipple between your thumb and forefinger, you will be able to check if there is any milk still in the breast.

- Never, ever allow your baby to suck on an empty breast; this will only lead to very painful nipples.

- If you find your baby is taking a lot less time than 30 minutes to feed, is happy and content until his feed and is gaining weight well, then you clearly have a very efficient feeder and there is no need to concern yourself if you finishes his feed much sooner than I suggest.

- Not all babies need the second breast in the early days. If your baby has totally emptied the first breast, burp him and change his nappy, then offer him the second breast. If he needs more he will take it. If not, start him off on that breast at the next feed.

- If your baby does feed from the second breast, you should still start on that breast at the next feed.

My methods for successful breast-feeding

The key to successful breast-feeding is getting off to the right start, and, as you will have already read, 'little and often' after the birth is essential to helping establish a good milk supply. But putting the baby to the breast little and often will not guarantee you a good milk supply if your baby is not positioned on the breast properly. While in the hospital you will be guided by your midwife and the nurses on how to latch your baby on to the breast. But as you will more than likely leave the hospital quite soon after giving birth, I would strongly advise that you get help from an experienced breast-feeding counsellor. There are several organisations which will arrange for someone to visit you in your home and spend time with you while you are feeding your baby to ensure that you are getting the positioning on the breast right. They will, if necessary, make several visits to you to help overcome any problems that you may encounter in the early days.

I would also highly recommend an excellent DVD by one of the leading breast-feeding counsellors in the country. Clare Byam-Cook, author of *What to Expect When You're Breast-feeding ... And What If You Can't?*, shows how to get to grips with breast-feeding in her DVD.

I advise all my mothers to start on day one by offering five minutes each side every three hours, increasing the time by a few minutes each day until the milk comes in. The three hours is calculated from the beginning of one feed to the beginning of the next feed. Somewhere between the third and fifth day, your milk will be in, and you should have increased the baby's sucking time on the breast to 15–20 minutes. Many babies will now be getting enough milk from the first breast, and be content to go three hours before needing a feed again. For example, if you start at 7pm the next feed will start at 10pm. However, if you find your baby is demanding food long before three hours have passed, he should of course be fed, and also offered both breasts at each feed, if he still remains unsettled. Once your milk is in, it is important that you make sure he has emptied the first breast totally before putting him to the second breast. In my experience mothers who change breasts too soon end up feeding their baby too much fore milk, which I believe is one of the main causes of babies never seeming satisfied and suffering from colic. It may take a sleepy baby 20–25 minutes to reach the very important hind milk (which is at least three times fattier than the fore milk) and to empty the breast.

Other babies may reach the hind milk much more quickly. Be guided by your baby as to how long he needs to get a good feed. If your baby feeds well, within the times I suggest, is happy and content between feeds and you are getting lots of wet nappies, he is obviously getting enough milk in the time he is on the breast.

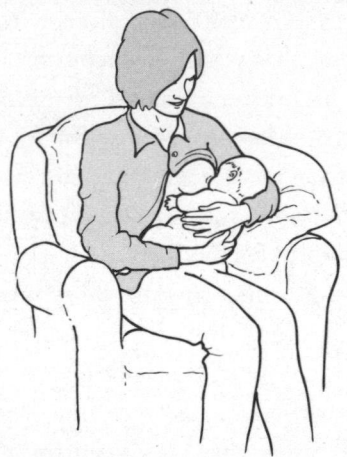

During the first few days, between 6am and midnight, wake your baby every three hours for short feeds. This will ensure that the feeding gets off to the best possible start in time for when the milk comes in. Feeding your baby three-hourly will help build up your milk supply much faster, and if he is fed enough during the day, your baby will be much more likely to go to sleep for longer periods between feeds in the night. It also avoids the mother becoming too exhausted, which, as I've said, is another major factor in breast-feeding going wrong. As with anything in life, success only comes from building a good foundation. All my mothers who establish three-hourly feeds in the hospital find that by the end of the first week a pattern has emerged. Then, very quickly, they can adapt their baby's feeding pattern to my first routine. The first breast-feeding routine (on page 164) not only helps you establish a good milk supply, but will also enable you to learn all your baby's many different needs: hunger, tiredness, boredom and overstimulation.

The main reasons my breast-feeding methods are so successful are:

- Feeding your baby three-hourly in the early days for shorter periods will gradually allow your nipples to get used to his sucking. It will also help ease the pain of engorgement when your milk comes in.

- Feeding little and often will help avoid the baby spending hours sucking on an empty breast trying to satisfy his hunger, which often occurs when a baby is allowed to go longer than three hours between feeds in the first week.

- A newborn baby's tummy is tiny and his needs can only be satisfied by feeding little and often. If you feed your baby three-hourly between 6am and midnight, the 'feeding all night syndrome' should never occur. Even if a very small baby is capable of going one longer spell in between feeds, following my advice ensures that this will happen to all babies at night and not during the day.

- Successful breast-feeding can only be achieved if a mother feels relaxed and comfortable. This is impossible if, having just given birth, you become exhausted from being awake and feeding all night.

- Newborn babies do not know the difference between day and night. Your baby will be able to learn the difference much sooner if you differentiate between daytime feeding and night-time feeding and do not allow him to sleep for long spells between feeds from 7am to 7pm.

Expressing

I believe that expressing milk in the early days plays a huge part in determining how successful a mother will be in breast-feeding while following a routine. I am convinced that one of the main reasons the majority of my mothers are so successful at breast-feeding is because I encourage the use of an electric expressing machine in the very early days.

The simple reason for this is that breast milk is produced on a supply and demand basis. During the very early days, most babies will empty the first breast and some may take a small amount from the second breast. Very few will empty both breasts at this stage. By the end of the second week, the milk production balances out and most mothers are producing exactly the amount their baby is demanding. Some time during the third and fourth week, the baby goes through a growth spurt and demands more milk. This is where a problem often sets in if you are attempting to put your baby into a routine and have followed the current advice of not expressing before six weeks.

In order to meet the increased demand for more food, you would more than likely have to go back to feeding two- or three-hourly and often twice in the night. This feeding pattern is repeated each time the baby goes through a growth spurt and often results in the baby being continually fed just prior to sleep time. This can create the problem of the wrong sleep association, making it even more difficult to get the baby back into the routine. Mothers who express the extra milk they produce in the very early days will always be producing more than their baby needs. When their baby goes through a growth spurt, the routine stays intact, because simply expressing less milk at the early-morning feeds can immediately satisfy any increased appetite. Expressing from the very early days can also help avoid the problem of a low milk supply. However, if your baby is over one month and you already have the problem of a low milk supply, by following my plan for increasing your milk supply (see page 313), you should see a big improvement within six days. For babies under one month, following the expressing times laid out in the routines should be enough to increase your supply. If you decide some time between one and four weeks to introduce a bottle (see page 73) of either expressed milk or formula at the late feed, you will be able to hand over feeding responsibility to someone else. This means that you will be able to get to bed early if you are feeling exhausted from night feeding. I advise in my routines that you express some milk at this time *or* that you feed the baby. If the baby takes a bottle, then you can express between 9.30–10pm and then go to bed. Expressing milk at this time is important to keep the supply going and ensure you have plenty for the middle-of-the-night feed.

If you have previously experienced difficulties with expressing, do not be disheartened. Expressing at the time suggested in my routines or the plan in Chapter 16 on common problems, along with the following guidelines, should help make it easier:

- The best time to express is in the morning as the breasts are usually fuller. Expressing will also be easier if done at the beginning of a feed. Express one breast just prior to feeding your baby, or feed your baby from one breast, then express from the second breast before offering him the remainder of his feed. Some mothers actually find that expressing is easier when done while they are feeding the baby on the other breast. It is also important to note that expressing at the beginning of a feed allows slightly longer for that breast to make more milk for the next feed. In my routines I suggest that the mother expresses at 6.45am; however, if you are producing a lot of milk and can't face the early-morning slot, you could move the expressing of the second breast to around 7.30am after the baby has fed from the first breast. A mother who is concerned about her milk supply or who is following the plan for increasing the milk (on page 313) should try to stick to the recommended times.

- In the early days, you may need to allow at least 15 minutes to express 60–90ml (2–3oz) at the morning feeds, and up to 30 minutes at the evening expressing times. Try to keep expressing times quiet and relaxed. The more you practise, the easier it will become. I usually find that, by the end of the first month, the majority of my mothers can easily express 60–90ml (2–3oz) within 10 minutes at the 9.30pm expressing when using a double pumping system.

- An electrical, heavy-duty pumping machine, the type used in hospitals, is by far the best way to express milk in the early days. The suction of these machines is designed to simulate a baby's sucking rhythm, encouraging the milk flow. If you are expressing both breasts at 9.30pm, it is worthwhile investing in an attachment that enables both breasts to be expressed at once, therefore reducing the time spent expressing.

- Sometimes, the let-down is slower in the evening when the breasts are producing less milk; a relaxing warm bath or shower will often help encourage the milk to flow more easily. Also, gently massaging the breasts before and during expressing will help.

- Some mothers find that it is helpful to have a picture of their baby close by for them to look at, while others find it better to watch a favourite television programme, or to chat to their partners. Experiment with different approaches to see which one works best for you.

As you proceed through the routines I advise which expressing times to drop. You cut back on expressing as your milk supply becomes firmly established. However, if you are returning to work I would recommend that you continue to express at the late feed until your baby is fully weaned at around six to seven months. Some mothers do find that their milk supply can reduce quite dramatically when they return to work, but continuing with the expressing will ensure that you keep your milk supply up. If you decide to wean before six months (after advice from a health professional) you can stop expressing straight away. If you have been advised to wean early, and once your baby is well established on three meals a day and has been consistently sleeping through 12 hours, you should be able to drop this expressing without it impacting on your milk supply.

Milk oversupply

One of the main reasons that I advise expressing in the early days is so that when the baby goes through a growth spurt, it ensures that his need for more milk is immediately met without a mother having to go back to giving extra feeds. It also ensures she will never have the problem of a low milk supply, which is one of the most common reasons why so many mother's give up breast-feeding. Although not so common, an oversupply of milk can sometimes also cause a problem with feeding. If you are fortunate enough to be one of those mothers who produces a lot more milk than your baby needs in the early weeks, then I would recommend that you do not follow the expressing times in the book, as this will only encourage your breasts to make even more milk and cause other problems with feeding.

If you are producing an excessive amount of milk you may find that you have problems with very full, engorged breasts, plugged ducts and mastitis. You may also feel intense pain when you have milk let-down. Another sign of oversupply is if you fully express and get more than 120–150ml (4–5oz) from one breast. If your baby weighs over 3.6kg (8lb) in weight, this should not be a problem as he would just continue to feed on the one breast at each feed until his appetite increases; however a baby who weighs less than that may rarely reach the hind milk and as a consequence suffer some of the problems below.

A baby whose mother is overproducing would show some or all of the following signs:

- Too much milk will often cause babies to fuss, pull off the breast, cry when feeding, pass lots of wind, possett excessively and have hiccups. They often want to feed more often on the breast, and perhaps gain weight more rapidly than the average baby (who usually gains 113–226g [4–8oz] each week during the first 3 or 4 months), or they may gain weight more slowly than the average baby.

- Their stools may be green and watery, and their bottoms may be red and sore. The mother's let-down reflex may be so forceful that the baby chokes, gags and sputters as he struggles with the jet of milk that sprays too quickly into his mouth.

- A baby who is only getting foremilk may be more prone to wind problems and spitting up as foremilk is higher in lactose.

> **Top Tips**
>
> Top tips to help you deal with an oversupply of milk:
>
> - Offer only one breast at each feed, and if he wants to feed again within an hour or so, then put him back on the same breast.
>
> - If you find that your let-down is very fast and your baby is getting upset when you put him to the breast, it's fine to express a very small amount off the breast before you feed him, but it is important not to express large amounts as this will only signal your breasts to produce even more milk.

- If he doesn't reach the hind milk at each feed, he will be missing out on the fats stored in it, and he would then demand to feed more quickly than if he has a feed of both foremilk and hind milk.

As your baby grows your milk supply will balance out to meet his needs and the problems of an oversupply will disappear. For further information on milk oversupply, please check out contentedbaby.com.

Breast-feeding and returning to work

If you are planning to return to work and would like to continue to breast-feed, it is important that you try to make sure that you have established a good milk supply, especially if you want your baby to have expressed breast milk during the day. A three-month-old baby could need two feeds of approximately 210–240ml (7–8oz) each of expressed milk if you are out between 9am and 5pm. As your baby will most likely be emptying both breasts at the 7am and 6pm feeds, you will need to express most of the milk for the feeds to be given in your absence during the working day and between 9pm and 10pm in the evening.

You should fit in two expressing sessions at around 10am and 2.30pm. If you express any later than this, it is possible that your breasts will not produce enough for the 6pm feed, especially if you are feeling tired.

The following guidelines give suggestions on how to incorporate working and breast-feeding:

- The longer you can spend at home establishing a milk supply, the easier it will be to maintain it once you return to work. Most breast-feeding experts advise a period of 16 weeks.

- Expressing from the beginning of the second week at the times suggested will enable you to build up a good stock of breast milk in the freezer.

- Introducing a bottle of expressed milk at the late feed by the second week will ensure that there will not be a problem of your baby not taking the bottle when you return to work.

- Check with your employer well in advance of returning to work that there will be a quiet place available where you will be able to express. Also check that they are happy for you to store the expressed milk in the refrigerator.

- Once you have established a good expressing routine using an electric expressing pump, you should begin to practise with a battery-operated one. With a single expressing pump you may find that switching from side to side throughout the expressing will help the milk to flow more easily. It may also be worthwhile considering a mini-electric pump that will enable you to express both breasts at once.

- Make sure that the nursery, or your nanny or childminder, is familiar with the storage and handling of breast milk, and how to defrost it.

- Establish the combined feeding routine that you will be using for your baby at least two weeks in advance of your return to work. This will allow you plenty of time to sort out any difficulties that may occur.

- Once you return to work, it is essential that you pay particular attention to your diet and that you rest well in the evening. It would be advisable to continue expressing at 9.30pm to ensure that you maintain a good milk supply. Also, make sure that you keep a good supply of breast pads at work, and a spare shirt or top!

Weaning your baby from the breast to the bottle

However long you have breast-fed for, it is important to plan the transition from breast-feeding to bottle-feeding properly. When deciding how long you intend to breast-feed your baby for, you should take into consideration that once you have established a good milk supply, you must allow approximately a week to drop each feed. For example, it can take six weeks to establish a good milk supply, and if you decide to give up breast-feeding, you should ideally allow, at the very least, a further five weeks to drop all breast-feeds and establish bottle-feeding. This information is very important for mothers who are planning to go back to work. If you give up breast-feeding before you have established a good milk supply, you should still allow enough time for your baby to get used to feeding from the bottle. Some babies can get very upset if they suddenly lose the pleasure and comfort they get from breast-feeding.

For a mother who has breast-fed for less than a month, I generally advise a period of 3–4 days in between dropping feeds. For a mother who has been breast-feeding longer than a month, it is best to allow 5–7 days in between dropping feeds. Assuming that the baby is already on a bottle-feed at the late feed, the next breast-feed to drop should be at 11am. The best way to do this is gradually to reduce the length of time the baby feeds from the breast by five minutes each day and top up with formula. Once your baby is taking a full bottle-feed, the breast-feed can be dropped. If you plan the weaning carefully from the breast to formula, your baby will have time to adjust to the bottle and you avoid the risk of developing mastitis. This can happen if the milk ducts become blocked due to engorgement, a common problem among mothers who instantly drop a feed.

I suggest that you continue to express at 9.30pm throughout the weaning process. The amount of milk expressed will be an indicator of how quickly your milk supply is going down. Some mothers find that once they are down to two breast-feeds a day, their milk reduces very rapidly. The signs to watch out for are your baby being irritable and unsettled after a feed, or wanting a feed long before it is normally due. If your baby shows either of these signs, he should be topped up immediately after the breast-feed with 30–60ml (1–2oz) of expressed milk or formula. This will ensure that his sleeping pattern does not go wrong due to hunger.

The chart opposite is a guideline for which feeds to drop first. Each stage represents the period of time between dropping feeds – either 3–4 days or 5–7 days, depending on how long you have been breast-feeding.

Time of feeds	7am	11am	2.30pm	6.30pm	9.30pm
Stage one	Breast	Formula	Breast	Breast	Express*
Stage two	Breast	Formula	Formula	Breast	Express
Stage three	Breast	Formula	Formula	Formula	Express
Stage four	Breast	Formula	Formula	Formula	
Stage five	Formula	Formula	Formula	Formula	

*I recommend that mothers should continue to express for the late feed (provided the baby is taking his bottle from his father or another helper) until the baby is 4–5 months old. This helps maintain a good milk supply, and can be used as an approximate gauge of how much milk they are producing. I find that a mother will usually produce overnight roughly twice the amount she has expressed. When you reach stage three of the weaning process, the 9.30pm expressing should be dropped gradually, reducing the expressing time by three minutes each night. Once you are only expressing 60ml (2oz) and going comfortably through the night, the expressing can be dropped altogether. When the last breast-feed has been dropped, care should be taken not to stimulate the breasts. Sitting in a warm bath with the water covering the breasts helps to get rid of any small amount of milk remaining in the breasts without stimulating them to make more.

Bottle-feeding

If you have decided to bottle-feed, the same routines as for breast-feeding should be followed. The only difference is that you may find your baby is happy to go longer than three hours after the 7am feed, otherwise the timing is exactly the same.

In the instances where a feed is being split – i.e. one breast before the bath and one after – the same pattern applies to bottle-feeding. I would normally make up two separate smaller feeds for this time.

How much and how often?

- Health authorities advise that a baby under four months would need 70ml (2½oz) of milk for each pound of body weight; for example, a baby weighing around 4.5kg (10lb) would need approximately 750ml (25oz) per day.

- This daily total would be divided between the number of feeds a day that the baby is taking. For example, a baby who is sleeping through the night may be having five feeds of around 150ml (5oz) a feed, whereas a baby still feeding in the night would be having six feeds of around 120ml (4oz) a feed.

- Babies who are being fed expressed milk from a bottle would have their individual feeds calculated in the same way, only they may not manage to go as long between feeds. Therefore, their daily milk intake could be slightly more than a formula-fed baby as they are fed more often.

- The feeding advice above is a guideline: hungrier babies may need an extra 30ml (1oz) at some feeds. If you have any concerns about the amount of milk your baby should be taking each day, it would be sensible to discuss it with your health visitor or GP.

Babies do not always drink the exact amount at each feed. Some feeds may be slightly bigger than others, so it's important to try to structure your feeds so he is taking the bigger feeds at the right times, i.e. 7am, 10.30am or 10.30pm. If you allow him to get into the habit of having bigger feeds in the middle of the night, it will eventually have the knock-on effect of him not being so hungry when he wakes in the morning. A vicious circle emerges where he needs to feed in the night because he does not feed enough during the day.

The same guidelines apply as for breast-feeding: aim to get the baby to take most of his daily milk requirements between 7am and 11pm. This way he will only need a small feed in the middle of the night, and will eventually drop it altogether. The chart below is an example of the feeding pattern of one of my babies during his first month. He weighed 3.2kg (7lb) at birth and, with a weekly gain of 180–240g (6–8oz), reached just over 4kg (9lb) when he was one month old. By structuring the feeding (the bigger feeds at the right times) he was well on the way to dropping his middle-of-the-night feed, and at six weeks he was sleeping through to 6.30am.

Times	7am	10–10.30am	2–2.30pm	5pm	6.15pm	10–11pm	2–4am	Total
Week 1	90ml	90ml	90ml	60ml	60ml	90ml	90ml	570ml
	(3oz)	(3oz)	(3oz)	(2oz)	(2oz)	(3oz)	(3oz)	(19oz)
Week 2	90ml	120ml	90ml	90ml	60ml	120ml	60ml	630ml
	(3oz)	(4oz)	(3oz)	(3oz)	(2oz)	(4oz)	(2oz)	(21oz)
Week 3	120ml	120ml	90ml	90ml	90ml	120ml	90ml	720ml
	(4oz)	(4oz)	(3oz)	(3oz)	(3oz)	(4oz)	(3oz)	(24oz)
Week 4	150ml	120ml	120ml	90ml	90ml	150ml	60ml	780ml
	(5oz)	(4oz)	(4oz)	(3oz)	(3oz)	(5oz)	(2oz)	(26oz)

N.B. These daily amounts of milk were calculated to suit that particular baby's needs. Remember to adjust the quantities of milk to suit your baby's own needs, depending on his weight (see page 74 on how to calculate the amount of milk your baby should be taking) but still follow the feeding times shown. During growth spurts make sure that the 7am, 10.30am and 10–11pm feeds are the first to be increased.

Establishing bottle-feeding

When your baby is born, the hospital may provide you with ready-made formula. You may be given a choice of two different brands; both are approved by the health authorities and there is very little difference in the composition of either milk. The bottles of formula will come with pre-packed sterilised teats, which are used once and then thrown away. Unless the jars have been stored in the fridge they do not need to be heated; they can be given at room temperature. However, if for some reason you do decide to heat the formula, do so by using either an electric bottle-warmer or by standing it in a jug of boiling water.

Never heat the formula in a microwave, as the heat may not be evenly distributed and you could end up by scalding your baby's mouth. Whichever form of heating you use, always test the temperature before giving the bottle to your baby. This can be done by shaking a few drops on the inside of your wrist; it should feel lukewarm, never hot. Once milk is heated, it should never be reheated, as this very rapidly increases the bacteria levels in the milk, which is one of the main causes of upset tummies in formula-fed babies. The advice given in hospital for formula-fed babies seems to be much the same as for breast-fed babies: 'Feed on demand whenever the baby wants and however much he wants.' While you do not have the problem of establishing a milk supply as in breast-feeding, many of the other problems are likely to occur. A bottle-fed baby weighing 3.2kg (7lb) or more at birth could go straight on to the one-to two-week routine, for example. A smaller baby might not manage to last quite as long between feeds and need feeding nearer three-hourly.

Ready-made formula is incredibly expensive to use all the time; most parents only use it on outings or in emergencies.

Before leaving the hospital, arrange for someone to buy at least two large tins of powdered formula milk of the same brand as the ready-made milk to which your baby has been introduced at the hospital. Make sure it is appropriate for newborns. It is no longer recommended that feeds be made up in advance. The NHS advises that the safest way to make up feeds is one at a time with water that has cooled to no lower than 70°C.

Hygiene and sterilisation

The utmost attention must be paid to hygiene: the sterilising of all your baby's feeding equipment and the preparation and storing of his formula milk.

The area where you sterilise and prepare your baby's formula should be kept spotlessly clean. Every morning the work-top should be thoroughly washed down with hot soapy water, the cloth used should then be rinsed well under hot running water and the surface wiped again to remove any traces of soap. This should be followed by a final wipe-down using kitchen roll and antiseptic spray.

The guidelines below, if applied to the letter, will reduce the risk of germs, which are so often the cause of tummy upsets in very young babies:

- Surfaces should be washed down thoroughly every day, as described above.

- After each feed the bottle and teat should be rinsed out thoroughly using cold water, and put aside in a bowl ready for washing and sterilising.

- Get into the habit of sterilising. Choose a time when you are not too tired and are able to concentrate properly. Most of my mothers find that 12 noon, when the baby has gone for his long nap, is a good time.

- Hands should always be washed thoroughly with anti-bacterial soap under warm running water, then dried with kitchen roll, not a tea towel, which is a breeding ground for germs.

- A separate kettle can be kept for boiling the baby's water; this avoids the water accidentally being boiled a second time if someone wants to make a cup of tea.

- Every day empty the kettle and rinse it out. The water from the tap should be allowed to run for a couple of minutes before filling the kettle.

- Fill the bowl in which the dirty bottles are stored with hot, soapy water. Using a long-handled bottle brush, carefully scrub all the bottles, rims, caps and teats inside and out. Particular attention should be given to the necks and rims. Carefully rinse everything under a running tap. Wash and rinse the bowl thoroughly, then place all the equipment in the bowl under the running hot water tap. This is to check that everything is thoroughly rinsed – the water should run clear.

- The steriliser should be rinsed out every day, and the removable parts checked and, if necessary, washed and rinsed. The bottles and teats should then be packed into the steriliser following the manufacturer's instructions.

- Refer to www.nhs.uk for current advice on how to make up formula.

Giving the feed

Prepare everything in advance: chair, cushions, bib and muslin. As with breast-feeding, it is important that you are sitting comfortably (see page 8), and in the early days I advise all mothers to support the arm in which they are holding the baby with a pillow, which enables you to keep the baby on a slight slope with his back straight. By holding the baby as shown in diagram A (below, top), you will lessen the likelihood of your baby getting air trapped in his tummy, which he might if fed as shown in diagram B.

● Before starting to feed, loosen and screw the teat back on; it should be very slightly loose. If it is screwed on too tightly it will not allow air into the bottle, and your baby will end up sucking and not getting any milk.

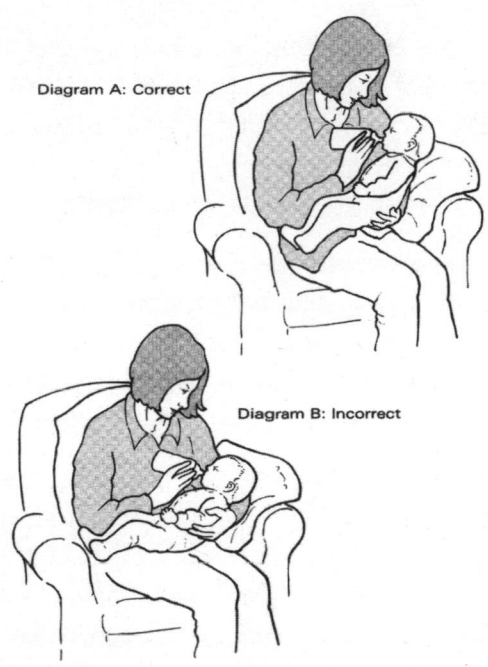

Diagram A: Correct

Diagram B: Incorrect

- Check also that the milk is not too hot; it should be just slightly warm. If you get your baby used to very warm milk, you will find that, as the feed progresses and the milk gets cool, he will refuse to feed. As it is dangerous to reheat the milk or keep it standing in hot water for any length of time, you could end up having to make up two bottles for every feed.

- Once feeding, make sure that the bottle is kept tilted up far enough to ensure that the teat is always filled with milk, to prevent your baby taking in too much air. Allow your baby to drink as much as he wants before stopping to burp him. If you try to burp him before he is ready he will only get very cross and upset.

- Some babies will take most of their feed, burp and then want a break of 10–20 minutes before finishing the remainder of the milk. In the early days, allowing for a break midway, it can take up to 40 minutes to give the bottle.

- Once your baby is 6–8 weeks old he will most likely finish his feed in about 20 minutes. If you find your baby is taking a very long time to feed, or keeps falling asleep halfway through a feed, it could be because the hole in the teat is too small. At this stage some babies are ready to go on to a faster flow teat.

- If your baby continues to feed very slowly and gets really fussy after taking only some of the feed, he might be ready to go longer between feeds. Although you may have to follow the correct routine for his age for sleeping, you might find that he is happy to follow the next routine for feeding.

- If you find that your baby is still getting fussy after only drinking a couple of ounces (60ml), it is better to give him a break in the middle of the feed than trying to cajole him to take all of his feed in one go. I have found that the easiest way to deal with feeding babies in this situation is to allow them to drink as much milk as they want and then not even attempt to offer them more for a further 20–30 minutes. I usually find they take the rest in about ten minutes, which is much better than spending a whole hour trying to get them to finish it.

- Occasionally, there are babies who will drink a full feed in 10–15 minutes and look for more. These babies are often referred to as 'hungrier babies'; the reality is that these babies are often 'sucky' babies, not hungrier ones. Because they have such a strong suck they are able to finish the bottle very quickly. Sucking is not only a means of feeding to a baby, but, in the early days, one of their natural pleasures. If your baby is taking the required amount of formula at each feed very quickly and looking for more, it may be worthwhile trying a teat with a smaller hole.

- Offering him a dummy after feeds may also help satisfy his 'sucking needs'. Remember a breast-fed baby is often sucking for 40 minutes or longer while feeding, so if your bottle-fed baby is feeding very quickly and getting fussy, it is worth considering a dummy in the early weeks to help him through this sucky stage. If you are unsure whether your baby is feeding enough for his size, it is worth having a discussion with your health visitor about the amount of milk he needs.

Successful bottle-feeding

It is very easy for bottle-fed babies to gain weight too quickly if they are allowed to have feeds in excess of the amounts recommended for their weight. While a few ounces a day should not create a problem, a baby who is overeating, and regularly putting on more than 240g (8oz) each week, will eventually become overweight and reach a stage where milk alone is not enough to satisfy his hunger. If this happens before the recommended age for giving solids, it can create a real problem. For establishing successful bottle-feeding the following guidelines should be observed:

- Before beginning the feed, check that the ring holding the teat and the bottle together is very slightly loose; if it is too tight it will restrict the flow of the milk.

- Check that the milk is the right temperature; it should be lukewarm, not hot.

- To avoid wind problems, which are very common among formula-fed babies, always make sure that you are comfortable and holding your baby correctly before beginning the feed.

- Some very young babies need a break in the middle of the feed, and if this is the case with your baby, you may have to allow up to an hour for him to take a full feed.

- If you find you are always having to wake your baby for the 7am feed, only to find he is not so hungry, then cut back the middle-of-the-night feed by 10ml every night until he is feeding better in the morning. It is really important not to cut back so much that he wakes up earlier in the morning.

- If you find that cutting back means he is back to waking twice in the night, I would advise that you continue to give your baby as much as he needs to get him through to 7am, accept for the time being that he only takes a small feed at this time, and then bring the next feed forward a little and top him up prior to the lunchtime nap.

- During growth spurts, make sure you follow the guidelines in the next section on which feeds to increase. This will avoid your baby cutting back, or even dropping, the wrong feeds first.

Formula: overfeeding

Unlike the breast-fed baby, the most common problem in the early days with formula-fed babies is overfeeding. The reason I believe this can happen with some babies is that they take the bottle of formula so quickly that their natural sucking instincts are not satisfied and they end up screaming when the bottle is removed from their mouth. Many mothers interpret this cry as one of hunger and end up giving them another bottle of formula. A pattern of overfeeding can quickly emerge, resulting in the baby gaining huge amounts of weight each week. If this problem is allowed to continue, the baby quickly reaches a stage where milk alone will not satisfy his appetite, yet he is too young to be given solids (under six months).

While it is normal for some babies to need an additional 30ml (1oz) at some feeds, special attention should be given if a baby is taking in excess of 150ml (5oz) every day, and is regularly gaining more than 240g (8oz) each week. When my formula-fed babies show signs of being particularly 'sucky', I have found that offering a dummy afterwards helps to satisfy their sucking needs. If you are concerned that your baby is overfeeding, it is essential that you discuss the problem with your health visitor or doctor.

Giving water to babies under six months

For many years it was recommended that a small drink of cool boiled water (around 30ml/1oz) could be offered to a baby aged between eight and twelve weeks who may be waking up at around 2–3am out of habit and not hunger. In my original books I only advised this if a baby took the water and then settled back to sleep for a couple of hours. Recently the advice on what age to give water has changed and it is recommended that babies are not given water before six months of age. If your baby is over six months of age and waking up in the night through habit and not hunger, it is fine to offer 30ml (1oz) or so of cool boiled water in the hope that he gets back to sleep. However, it is pointless to keep offering water at this time if you baby refuses to settle back to sleep quickly or wakes up again after 30–40minutes. If you persist with offering water over several nights with an unsettled baby, you will actually be encouraging your baby to sleep badly in the night, which is the opposite of what you really want. Night feeds are easier to eliminate when a baby feeds quickly and settles back to sleep until the morning, than a baby who is awake on and off during the night being offered water, the dummy or cuddles to get back to sleep. However, it is important also to look at your baby's daytime feeding and improve on that so he does not wake up in the night due to genuine hunger.

Diluting feeds

It has been common practice for many years among some health advisors to dilute middle-of-the-night feeds in order to get the baby to drop the feed as quickly as possible. I do not recommend diluting formula feeds for babies under the age of six months. If babies older than six months are feeding excessively in the night, diluting the feed should only be done on the advice of a GP or pediatrician. Diluting feeds can be dangerous and has been known to result in death. If you feel your baby is waking in the night not due to genuine hunger, but out of habit, then a very small feed and a cuddle should get him back to sleep quickly until nearer 6–7am. If he does not settle with a small feed and a cuddle, then he should be offered a big enough feed so that he sleeps nearer to 6–7am. It is important not to restrict the feed so much in the night that he wakes a second time around

5–6am.The aim of the CLB routines should always be get your new baby feeding once in the night, and sleeping near to 7am. In order to achieve this your baby must be given enough milk in the middle of the night to sleep to 7am. If not, you could possibly end up with an early morning waking problem. It is also important, before looking to eliminate feeds in the night, to check that your baby is taking near the recommended amount of formula for his weight.

Your questions answered

Q I have very small breasts and am worried that I may not be able to produce enough milk to satisfy my baby's needs.

- Breast size is totally irrelevant when it comes to producing breast milk. Each breast, regardless of shape or size, has 15–20 ducts, each duct with its own cluster of milk-making cells. Milk is made within these cells and pushed down the ducts when the baby sucks.

- During the early days, make sure your baby is put to the breast frequently. Most babies need a minimum of eight feeds a day to help stimulate the breasts and establish a good milk supply.

- Always make sure that your baby totally empties the first breast before putting him on the second breast. This signals the breast to make more milk and also ensures that your baby gets the important hind milk.

Q My friend was in agony when her milk came in. Is there anything I can do to help relieve the pain of engorgement?

- Put your baby to the breast often and do not let him go longer than three hours during the day between feeds or 4–5 hours at night.

- A warm bath or warm wet flannels placed on the breasts before a feed will help the milk flow and, if need be, gently expressing a little milk by hand will make it easier for the baby to latch on.

- Damp flannels chilled in the fridge and placed on the breasts after a feed will help constrict the blood vessels and reduce the swelling.

- Take the leaves just under the outer leaves of a cabbage, chill in the fridge and place on your breasts inside your bra between feeds.

- Wear a well-fitting nursing bra that supports your breasts. Make sure that it is not too tight under the arms and does not flatten your nipples.

Q Many of my friends had to give up breast-feeding because it was so painful.

- The main reason women experience pain in the early days is because the baby is not positioned on the breast correctly. The baby ends up chewing on the end of the nipple, causing much pain for the mother, more often than not resulting in cracked, bleeding nipples and a poor feed for the baby. A pattern soon emerges of the baby needing to feed again very quickly, giving him even more opportunity to damage the nipples.

- Make sure that you always hold your baby with his tummy to your tummy and that his mouth is open wide enough for him to take all of the nipple and as much of the areola as he can manage into his mouth.

- Apart from ensuring that your baby is well positioned, it is important that you are sitting comfortably. The ideal chair should have a straight back, preferably with arms so that you can position a cushion to support the arm in which you are holding the baby (see page 8). If you do not support your arm, it will be much more difficult to position and support your baby properly. This can cause him to pull on the breast, which will be painful for you.

Q I have a three-week-old baby and am getting very concerned over the conflicting advice. Some people say give both breasts at each feed, others say one is enough.

- Be guided by your baby. If he feeds from one breast, is content to go three hours between feeds, and is gaining weight steadily each week, one breast is obviously enough. Please remember that the three hours goes from the beginning of one feed to the beginning of the next feed.

- If he is looking for food after two hours, or is waking up in the night more than once, it would be advisable to offer him the second breast. You may find he only needs the second breast later in the day when your milk supply is at its lowest.

- Whether your baby has one or two breasts at a feed, always check that the first breast is completely empty before putting him on the second. This can be done by gently squeezing the area around the nipple between your thumb and forefinger.

Q Do I need to avoid certain foods while breast-feeding?

- You should continue with the same varied, healthy diet that you followed throughout your pregnancy. In addition, you should include small healthy snacks between meals to help keep your energy levels up.

- Ensure that you eat plenty of protein either poultry, lean meat, fish. Vegetarians and vegans should eat the equivalent in beans, pulses and grains, etc. I have noticed that on the days when some of my breast-feeding mothers did not eat enough protein, their babies were much more unsettled.

- Some research points to dairy products as the cause of colic in certain babies. If you find your baby develops colic, it may be wise to discuss how to monitor your dairy intake with your health visitor or paediatrician.

- Artificial sweeteners and caffeine should be avoided. Remember that caffeine is not only found in coffee, but also in tea, soft drinks and chocolate. I have found all of these things can upset most babies.

- Strawberries, tomatoes, mushrooms, onions and fruit juice, if taken in large quantities, have left many of my babies very irritable. While I do not suggest cutting out these from your diet, I would suggest that you keep a record of any food or drink consumed 12–16 hours prior to your baby showing signs of tummy ache, explosive bowel movements, excessive wind and crying fits.

- While working in the Middle East and Far East, I observed that breast-feeding mothers followed a much blander diet than normal, and that highly spiced foods were omitted from their diet. Perhaps it would be wise to avoid very spicy food in the early days.

Q My two-week-old baby wakes up yelling for a feed, only to fall asleep after five minutes on the breast. He then demands to be fed two hours later, leaving me absolutely exhausted.

- Always make sure your baby is fully awake before you attempt to feed him. Unwrap him in the cot, take his legs out of his baby-grow and allow the cool air to get to his skin, and give him time to wake up by himself. Then you can start his feed.

- It is very important that sleepy babies are kept cool while feeding. He should not be overdressed and the room should not be too warm. Have a play mat next to you on the floor and the minute he gets sleepy, put him on it. If necessary, remove his baby-grow, as this will encourage him to stretch and kick. Within a few minutes he will probably protest about being put down, so pick him up and give him a few more minutes on the same breast. This procedure often has to be repeated two or three times. Once he has had 20 minutes on the first breast, burp him well and change his nappy. He can then be put back on the first breast if he has not emptied it, or transferred to the second.

- If possible, get your partner to do the late feed with expressed milk. This way, you will at least manage to get an uninterrupted few hours' sleep for one part of the night.

Q My son is 16 weeks old. Over the last two weeks he has become increasingly difficult to feed. He dropped the middle-of-the-night feed at around 11 weeks old yet, despite not feeding after the late feed, he is fairly disinterested in his 7am feed, taking as little as 60ml (2oz). He then cries on and off until I feed him at 11am. When I feed him earlier than 11am he then does not sleep well at lunchtime, waking up after an hour

looking for a feed. When I feed him then, it puts the rest of the feeds out for the afternoon.

- To get your son more interested in his 7am feed, try cutting back on his late feed. Although he will need a small feed at this time, probably until he is weaned on to solids, try reducing it gradually to 90–120ml (3–4oz) and see if he is more interested at 7am. If this helps him feed better at 7am then continue to reduce the amount he takes then to 90–120ml (3–4oz).

- If you find that by cutting back on the late feed your son starts to wake up earlier in the morning, I would recommend that you go back to giving him more at the late feed and accept that for a short while he will only take a smaller feed in the morning. This is better than him waking up earlier and needing to be fed again in the night.

- Until he is feeding better at 7am you will have to feed him earlier than 11am, possibly by 10.15am, but I would suggest that you top him up around 11.15–11.30am to ensure that he has taken enough milk to ensure he sleeps well at his lunchtime nap.

- You may also find that when he goes through a growth spurt he starts to take his morning bottle much more quickly and may even start waking up earlier, looking for a feed. When this happens I would suggest that you go back to giving him more at the late feed to ensure he gets through to 7am. You may have to do this for a week or so, and perhaps even continue with a larger feed until he is weaned. However, if he started to get fussy about the morning feed again, you would then have to cut back on the late feed once more.

4

Understanding Your Baby's Sleep

Sleep is probably the most misunderstood and confusing aspect of parenthood. The misconception is that for the first few weeks all the baby will do is feed and sleep. While many do, the fact that there are so many sleep consultants in the United Kingdom for babies and children is proof that a great many do not. If your newborn or young baby is one of the latter – tense, fretful and difficult to settle – please take heart, as this need not be a reflection of your baby's future sleep habits.

The majority of babies that I helped care for personally usually started to sleep to 6–7am from the late feed somewhere between eight and twelve weeks. A few slept through before that age and some still needed to be fed in the night for much longer. As I do not know your baby personally, I cannot give you a specific answer as to when he will sleep through, as many factors will dictate that. For example, if your baby was born prematurely or you did not start following the routines until he was several weeks old, then obviously he may take longer to sleep through the night. The important thing to remember is that what you are trying to achieve in the early days is a regular sleeping pattern, where your baby settles well in the evening, feeds and settles after the late feed, and then only wakes once in the night for a feed and goes back to sleep quickly until 6–7am.

The aim of the routines is to achieve this without causing distress to you or your baby; they are not about pushing your baby through the night at the earliest possible age without feeding him. By following the guidelines I have laid out in this book, and adjusting the routines if need be to suit your baby's own particular needs, he will sleep the longest spell at night as soon as he is physically and mentally capable of doing so. The key to achieving this is to be patient, consistent and allow time for my routines to become established. Once they are, you can avoid the agony of months of sleepless nights that so many parents go through. It has worked for hundreds of thousands of babies and their parents, so it can work for you!

If you want your baby to sleep through the night from an early age and ensure a long-term healthy sleep pattern, the golden rules are to establish the right associations, and to structure your baby's feeds from the day you arrive home from the hospital. The ideal is that your baby takes most of his nutritional needs in the form of milk during the day. If you allow your baby to miss a daytime feed because he is sleeping too much, his tummy is too small to take extra at the next feed so he will then need to feed more in the night.

The advice given in many of the baby books, and by some hospital staff, is that newborn babies should feed on demand for as often and for as long as they need. You will be told to accept that your baby's erratic sleeping and feeding patterns are normal and that things will improve by three months of age. Since the publication of my first book in 1999, I have received thousands of phone calls, emails and letters from distraught parents whose infants, aged anywhere between three months and three years, have serious sleep and feeding problems. This continually disproves the theory that babies will put themselves into a routine by three months. Even if a baby does do this, it is unlikely to be a routine that fits in with the rest of the family.

While some experts agree that some babies are capable of sleeping through the night by three months, they do not stress the importance of guiding the baby towards this goal. The innocent and weary parent believes in and hopes for a miraculous improvement at three months, but this is unlikely to happen if baby has not learned the difference between day and night, naps and the long sleep, and if the parent has not learned how to structure feeds, which needs to be established from day one. Ensuring that your baby feeds little and often during the day is essential if you want to avoid his waking up genuinely hungry every couple of hours during the night.

Since starting my consultancy service for new parents I have received many desperate calls from the maternity wards. The cry for help is nearly always the same. The baby is feeding for up to an hour at a time, usually two-hourly from 6pm until 5am. The mother is often exhausted and starting to suffer from cracked nipples.

When I ask what the baby is like during the day the usual reply is: 'He's ever so good during the day; he will feed, then go four hours or longer.'

It continues to baffle me that such contradictory advice is still being given to new parents. They are told that it is normal for a newborn baby to need to feed as much as 8–12 times in a 24-hour period, but they should then allow the baby to sleep hours between daytime feeds. It is hardly surprising that a baby who has had only four or even fewer feeds between 6am and 6pm is going to wake up many times in the night to satisfy his daily needs. This is one of the main reasons that I am opposed to the advice that babies should be demand fed. It does not take into account that many babies do not demand to be fed in the early days.

Sleep and demand-feeding

The phrase 'demand-feeding' is used time and time again, misleading a mother into believing that any sort of routine in the early days could deny her baby nutritionally and, according to some experts, emotionally. While I would totally agree that the old-fashioned four-hourly routine of feeding, whether breast or bottle, is not natural to newborn babies, I feel the term 'feeding on demand' is used too loosely.

The pattern for sleepless nights is unfortunately often set before mother and baby leave the hospital. Because the baby has been allowed to sleep for long spells between feeds during the day, he genuinely needs to feed on and off all evening and every couple of hours in the night. A vicious circle soon emerges where the baby is sleeping for most of the day because he has been awake most of the night. This type of sleeping and feeding pattern is encouraged by many experts as they believe that the baby should take the lead where feeding is concerned. Hence the terms 'baby-led feeding' or 'demand-feeding'. Some experts even go as far as to say that it is 'damaging' to wake a sleeping baby, and take a very hostile view of my advice to do so. It was my experience of working with many sets of twins and premature babies that helped me to realise this was complete nonsense. I observed that when I went to care for these babies, the hospital staff had already implemented a feeding routine. Because the lives of these tiny, sleepy babies depended on being fed little and often, they would not have dared take the risk of allowing them to go long spells between feeds. This experience went a long way in helping me develop the CLB routines. Contrary to what some people try to imply, the routines are not about denying the baby food, but about ensuring that they are fed enough. As I have already mentioned, I have had personal experience of caring for babies who nearly lost their lives due to dehydration, because they were not demanding to be fed enough. This further convinced me that demand-feeding puts a baby at much more risk than if the baby is woken at regular intervals and offered a feed.

Because breast milk is produced on a supply and demand basis – i.e. the breasts make the amount of milk that the baby demands – within a few weeks the demand-fed baby often starts to demand to be fed two-hourly not only at night but during the day as well. This is because the feeding pattern of the previous 2–3 weeks has affected the supply of breast milk. Because the baby is feeding so often it is inevitable that, more often than not, the baby is being fed to sleep. This can often lead to long-term sleeping problems for many babies.

After months of sleepless nights and exhausting days with the baby still feeding two- or three-hourly, many parents ask their GP to refer them to a baby sleep clinic. Or they purchase one or several of the many baby books on how to get your baby to sleep through the night, only to be told they got it all wrong in the first place. The real reason their baby is unable to sleep well is that he has had the wrong associations with going to sleep, i.e. feeding, rocking, patting, etc.

How well your baby sleeps is very closely linked to how well he feeds, and what he associates with falling asleep. To encourage healthy sleep habits with your baby, it is important that you not only structure his feeding but you have an understanding of the sleep rhythms of young babies, so that you establish the right sleep associations from very early on.

An understanding of sleep rhythms will also help you adjust the routines to suit the individual needs of your baby and, at times, on the occasions when it has not been possible to follow them to the letter.

Sleep rhythms

Most of the leading experts would agree that a newborn baby will sleep approximately 16 hours a day in the first few weeks. This sleep is broken up into a series of short and longer sleeps. In the early days sleep is very much linked to the baby's need to feed little and often. It can take well up to an hour to feed, burp and change the baby, after which time he falls quickly into a deep sleep. If the baby has fed well he will often sleep through to the next feed. Over a 24-hour period, therefore, with the baby feeding 6–8 times a day and feeds lasting between 45 minutes and one hour, the baby ends up sleeping approximately 16 hours a day. However, between the third and fourth week, the baby becomes more alert and will not fall straight into a deep sleep after feeding. This is often a time when things start to go wrong and the wrong sleep associations are developed. The anxious parents, believing that the baby should fall asleep straight after feeding, start to resort to feeding, rocking or giving the baby a dummy to induce sleep. They do not realise that it is around this age that the different stages of sleep become more apparent. Like adults, babies drift from light sleep into a dream-like sleep known as REM sleep, then into a deep sleep. The cycle is much shorter than that of an adult, lasting approximately 30–40 minutes. While some babies only stir when they drift into light sleep, others will wake up fully. If the baby is due a feed, this does not create a problem. However, if it is only one hour since the baby fed, and the baby does not learn to settle himself, a real problem can develop over the months ahead if the baby is constantly assisted back to sleep by one or more of the methods I have just mentioned. Recent research has shown that all babies drift into light sleep and wake up approximately the same number of times during the night. Only the poor sleepers are unable to drift back into deep sleep, because they are used to being helped to sleep. If you want your baby to develop good sleep habits from an early age, it is important to avoid the wrong sleep associations. My routines are structured so that your baby feeds well, never gets overtired and does not learn the wrong associations when going to sleep.

The bedtime routine

Once your baby has regained his birth weight and is gaining weight steadily, you can look at establishing a regular bedtime of 6.30–7pm, and allow him to sleep past the 9pm feed, feeding him at around 10pm instead, slowly pushing forwards to 10.30pm. It is also at this stage that he should manage to go slightly longer in the night. If he feeds well at this feed, and settles at around 11–11.30pm, he will hopefully manage to sleep to between 2–3am. If he feeds well then and hopefully settles back within an hour, he should manage to sleep to around 6–7am, provided that he has been awake properly enough to take a full feed at the late feed. During the early days, how soon they wake up after midnight is very much dependent on how awake they were at the late feed and how much they took. It is worthwhile spending some time at this feed to ensure that the baby does start to sleep a longer stretch in the night.

Establishing a good bedtime routine and getting your baby to sleep well between 7–10pm is a major factor in how quickly he will sleep through the night. A baby who feeds well at 6pm, and settles to sleep well between 7pm and 10pm, will wake up refreshed and ready to take a full feed. However, there are other factors in establishing a regular bedtime routine. The main ones are that you have structured his feeding and sleeping pattern during the day, so that he is hungry enough to take a full feed at 5–6.15pm; and that he has been awake enough during the day, so he is ready to sleep at 7pm.

I get many calls and emails from parents who are struggling to settle their babies in the evening. When a pattern of feeding on and off occurs during the evening, in most cases it has a knock-on effect of the baby not being hungry enough at the late feed. The baby then ends up waking around 1am and usually 4–5am again, genuinely hungry.

Establishing a bedtime routine will only be possible if your baby is well-fed and ready to sleep by 6.30–7pm. For example, if you allow your baby to sleep for lengthy periods in the late afternoon, he is unlikely to settle well at 7pm, even if he has fed well. The key to encouraging your baby to sleep well at night is very dependent on what happens during the day.

Once he is gaining weight steadily, it means he is growing well. As he grows, the amount that he can take at each feed should increase, and he should gradually be able to go longer between some feeds. Ideally, this longer spell should be between 7pm and 10pm, and after the late feed and middle-of-the-night feeds. This will not necessarily happen automatically, which takes us back to what you may find the hardest part of the routines: waking your baby for daytime feeds at the recommended times for his age. But it is simply common sense that if your baby has fed regularly during the day, he should, as he grows, need to feed less in the night, as the amount that he takes during the day increases.

Try, whenever possible, to start the day at 7am, stick to the times I advise in the routines, and ensure that your baby takes a full feed at those times and is awake for short spells after the daytime feeds. This will help you establish a bedtime routine where your baby settles well at 7pm.

Remember, if your baby feeds and settles well by 7pm and sleeps soundly until the late feed, he will be much more likely to start to sleep longer in the night after that feed, provided that he has been awake enough to take a full feed.

As very young babies get overtired easily, start the bedtime routine no later than 6pm. If your baby has not slept well at nap times you may need to start earlier. Try to keep things very calm and quiet throughout the bath, and after the bath avoid lots of eye contact and talking, so that he does not become overstimulated.

Try always to do the last part of the feed in a quiet, dimly lit room, so that you can quickly settle your baby in his bed before he falls into a deep sleep.

It isn't always easy, and takes great perseverance, especially if you are getting pressure to go with the flow from well-meaning family and friends. All the parents I have spoken to say that it was worth putting in the hard work in those early days, as their babies started to sleep longer and longer in the night, until they eventually make it through to that magical time of 7am.

Here are my tips for ensuring your baby settles well at 7pm, then in turn feeds well at the late feed so he sleeps the longest spell at night:

- During the day ensure that your baby stays awake as near as possible to the recommended times for his age (see page 162).

- In the early days some babies may need to be settled in the bed by 6.30pm.

- If your baby is not settling well at bedtime, check that the possible cause is not hunger by offering him a top-up of expressed milk or, if bottlefed, an extra ounce of formula.

- When feeding your baby try to do so sitting in a chair as near to his bed as possible, therefore he will not become too aroused when transferred from your arms to his bed.

- Once you have fed your baby try to burp him in the sitting up position rather than over your shoulder. When babies are due to go to sleep they can quickly fall asleep on the shoulder and this often results in the baby getting upset the minute they are put in their bed. This is because when you lay him flat in his bed he will immediately miss the pressure on his tummy and the comfort that he feels when he is lying over your shoulder.

Early-morning waking

I have always believed that whether a child becomes an early-morning waker is very much determined by what happens during the first year. In order to avoid this problem it is crucial that the baby sleeps at night in a very dark room and that the mother treats any feeds before 7am as night-time feeds. They should be done with the minimum of fuss, with no talking or eye contact, and the baby should be settled back to sleep until 7am. If your baby has woken between 6am and 6.30am, and is less than two months old, then leave him until 7.30am. If he is over two months old I would advise that you wake him up by 7.15am. When adding up your baby's daily naptime, remember that any sleep just after 7am or prior to 7pm should be included in the daily recommended amount of sleep for his age. This approach has worked for the hundreds of babies I have helped care for, none of whom ever got up before 7am, once they were sleeping through the night. Certainly some of these babies would waken around 5–6am, and perhaps chatter or sing for a short spell, before returning to sleep.

Since the publication of the first edition of this book I have spoken to thousands of parents who have experienced problems with early-morning waking, and a further reason has become very apparent. One thing that nearly all these parents had in common is that they did not follow my advice of allowing their babies to wake up naturally. Most admitted to picking their babies up the minute they started to wake from daytime naps. Over a period of time it is not surprising that these babies came to expect the same thing to happen when they woke early in the morning. Somewhere between eight and twelve weeks, the majority of babies do not wake up from naps immediately looking for food. This is a good time to encourage them to lie in their cot for a short time after waking. I am convinced that by doing this, along with the guidelines listed below, there will be less chance of your baby becoming an early-morning waker:

- Research shows that the chemicals in the brain work differently in the dark, preparing it for sleep. From six months, when your baby can be put to sleep in his nursery, check that there are no chinks of light at the top or sides of the curtains or round the door. Even the smallest amount of light can be enough to wake the baby fully when he comes into a light sleep. It would be worth investing in blackout lining for the nursery, as well as for your bedroom where he will sleep at night for the first six months.

- Until they reach six months the 'Moro reflex' can be quite strong with some babies and is very obvious in the early days. The baby flings his arms and legs back in jerky movements, usually if he gets shocked, is startled by a sudden loud noise or is put down too roughly or too quickly. Hence the reason that it is often referred to as the 'startle reflex'. For this reason I believe it is very important that a baby is tucked in very securely by his bed covers, until the Moro reflex has totally disappeared. The sheet and blankets should be placed lengthways across the width of the cot and then two rolled hand towels pushed down between the spars and the mattress. For babies who still manage to work their way up the cot, a very lightweight sleeping bag of no more than 0.5 tog can be used, along with being tucked in with a cotton sheet.

- Do not try to push your baby through the night by cutting down on his middle-of-the-night feed. Continue to give him as much as he wants in the middle of the night to ensure that he sleeps soundly to 7am. It is only when he has been sleeping through regularly to 7am for a period of time, and wakes up refusing to feed well at 7am, that you should consider slowly reducing the amount he is taking in the middle of the night.

- If your baby is feeding at 5–6am, treat it as a night feed. It should be done as quickly as possible in a dimly lit room without any eye contact or talking. Only change his nappy if really necessary. It is important that you offer him as much as he wants so that he sleeps nearer to 7am. There is no point in restricting this feed, if he then wakes up again at 6.30am.

- If your baby feeds between 5am and 6am he will obviously need to be topped up around 8am. Because he has already fed earlier this top up may be quite a small one, which will mean he could be hungry earlier for his next feed. I often find that until a baby is sleeping nearer to 7am he will sometimes need a split feed between 5–6am and 7.30–8am, and then again around 10–10.30am and 11.30am–12pm. Do not feel that this is a back track; the main reason for splitting the feeds is to ensure that he takes enough milk to settle well for his lunch time nap and get him back on track. Once he sleeps to nearer 7am, you can then go back to giving him one feed then and another one around 11am, although if a baby is not sleeping well at lunch time I advise offering a top-up just prior to the lunch time nap.

- I recommend that the late feed should not be dropped until the baby is well-established on solids food, which can be anywhere between six and seven months. The reason being that if he goes through a growth spurt before he start solids, he can be offered extra milk at this feed, to ensure that he does not wake up early due to hunger.

- If you find that your baby is absolutely refusing to feed at the late feed or is waking up an hour or so later after taking only a small feed, then you probably will have no choice but to drop it. It is pointless being up in the night two or three times giving small feeds. However, if you do decide to drop the feed you may find that for a few weeks your baby will feed twice in the night between midnight and 7am. For example, if he feeds at midnight, he will possibly wake again around 4 or 5am again and genuinely need to feed. It is very rare that a baby will sleep until midnight and then sleep a further six hours after being fed at midnight. I have had some that did do that, but they are certainly in the minority. Also when dropping the late feed it is important not to restrict the amount of milk that he does take when he wakes. I say that the majority of babies once they reach three to four months, should manage to sleep a longer stretch of eight to nine hours, from the late feed to nearer 6–7am. Therefore if you drop the late feed around this age, he is not being unreasonable to wake up and need a feed eight to nine hours later, perhaps around 3–4am in the morning. Once solids are introduced and he is well established on three meals a day, he should then gradually start to sleep later until he is sleeping from 7pm to 6–7am.

Your questions answered

Q How many hours' sleep a day does my newborn baby need?

- Depending on weight and whether the baby was premature, most babies need approximately 16 hours a day, broken up into a series of short and long sleeps.

- Smaller babies and premature babies tend to need more sleep, and will be more likely to doze on and off between feeds.

- Larger babies are capable of staying awake for an hour or so and sleeping for at least one longer spell of 4–5 hours during a 24-hour period.

- By the age of one month, most babies who are feeding well and gaining weight steadily are capable of sleeping for one longer stretch of 5–6 hours from the late feed.

Q How do I make sure that the longer stretch of sleeping is always in the night and not during the day?

- Follow my routines and always start your day no later than 7am, so that you can fit in all the feeds before 11pm.

- Try to keep your baby awake for at least 6–8 hours between 7am and 7pm.

- Ensure that your baby stays awake for as much of the two-hour social period as possible. Once he is awake for a total of eight hours between 7am and 7pm, he will be more likely to sleep longer in the night.

- Always distinguish between sleep and awake time. During the first few weeks, ensure the area where your baby is sleeping is kept as quiet as possible.

- Do not overstimulate your baby with lots of talking or eye contact during the feeds between 7pm and 7am.

Q I am trying to stick to your routines, but my four-week-old baby can only stay awake for an hour at the most after feeds. Should I be trying to make him stay awake longer?

- If your baby is feeding well and gaining weight steadily, sleeping well between feeds in the night and is alert for some of his awake periods during the day, he is just one of those babies who needs more sleep.

- If he is waking up more than twice in the night or staying awake for over an hour in the night despite feeding well at the late feed, try stimulating him a bit more during the day.

- While the late feed should always be a quiet feed, in my experience a baby under three months needs to be awake for at least 45 minutes. I found that too sleepy a feed at this time usually resulted in the baby being more awake around 2–3am, or waking up at 2am and 5am. Although it can be tempting to do a late sleepy feed, I think that the effort put into having the baby properly awake at this times usually pays off with them sleeping through the night much quicker than if they are hardly awake at this time.

- If you structure your baby's feeds and sleep times between 7am and 11pm by my routines, when your baby does cut back his sleep, it will be at the right time.

Q The routine seems very restricting. If I go out with my four-week-old during waking time he goes straight to sleep in the buggy, which means he has slept too much.

- Whether your baby is in my routine or not, during the first couple of months life is restrictive due to the amount of time spent feeding.

- By two months most babies are capable of going longer between feeds and are quicker at feeding. This makes outings easier.

- For the first two months if you plan your outings to fit around his sleep time, by eight weeks he will be able to stay awake longer when you take him out in the car or buggy.

Q My four-week-old baby has suddenly started to wake up at 9pm. If I feed him then he wakes up twice in the night at 1am and 5am. I have tried encouraging him to hold out until 10.30pm, but then he is so tired he doesn't feed properly, which means he still wakes up earlier.

- Around one month, the light and deep sleep becomes much more defined. I find that a lot of babies come into a very light sleep around 9pm, so ensure that the area around where your baby is sleeping is kept as quiet as possible.

- Breast-fed babies may need a top-up of expressed milk after the 6pm feed.

- If you have to feed him at 9pm, try to settle him back to sleep with one breast or a couple of ounces (60 ml), and then push the 10.30pm feed to 11.30pm. Hopefully, he will then take a full feed, which would get him through to 3.30am.

- Alternatively, try giving a split feed. Offer your baby a feed at 9.30pm and then keep him awake until you offer a further feed at 10.30pm.

Q I always have to wake my baby of 10 weeks for his late feed, then he only takes 90–120ml (3–4oz) and wakes again at 4am. Could I just drop the last feed and see if he goes through until 4am without that feed?

- I would not advise getting rid of the feed yet, as he could wake up at 1am and then 5am, which, in effect, would be two night wakings. I have always found it best to get the baby sleeping through to 7am, and taking solids, before dropping the late feed. This usually happens at about six months.

- To encourage your baby to drink more at the late feed and sleep longer in the night it may be worth introducing a split feed at the late feed. For this to work well you should start to wake your baby at around 9.45pm, so he is fully awake and feeding by 10pm. Allow him to drink as much of the feed as he would want, then allow him a good kick on the floor on his play mat. At 11pm you should then take him to the bedroom and change his nappy, then offer him a further feed. If you are formula-feeding I would advise that you make a fresh feed up for the second feed.

5

Establishing the Contented Little Baby Routines

The times for feeding and sleeping change 10 times during the first year of the CLB routines to ensure that the individual needs of every baby can be properly met. It is very important that you carefully read the advice and information in the feeding and sleeping chapters before you even attempt to start the routines. They will help you understand how best to use the routines so that your baby is happy, content and feeds and sleeps well. After the birth follow the advice given for a newborn, until he has regained his birth weight and shows signs of being able to go longer between feeds. Then you can move on to the first routine. Gradually, when your baby shows signs of going longer between feeds and staying awake longer, you can move on to the next routine. Do not worry if your baby is not managing the routine for his age, just stick to the routine that he is happy in and continue to watch for the signs that he is content and able to go longer between feeds and stay awake longer, before moving on to the next routine.

Feeding

Small babies spend a great deal of their waking time feeding. To avoid excessive night feeding, it is important to structure and establish a good daytime feeding pattern. As I have explained,

Top Tips

If you are starting the routines with an older baby who has established a pattern of demand-feeding and sleeping, look through the routines and find the one nearest to the pattern he is already in. Follow this for a short period and then, once he is eating and feeding happily at the correct times, you can move on to the next routine, gradually working your way through the different routines until he eventually reaches the one suitable for his age.

in order to establish a good milk supply I believe that your baby needs to be fed little and often after the birth. The success of the CLB routines depends on the baby being woken for feeds and not being left for long spells between feeds. I recommend that in the very early days a three-hourly feeding routine be established. This time is calculated from the beginning of one feed to the beginning of the next feed. Of course, if a baby is demanding food before the recommended time I have always advised that he should be fed. But if this continues long after the milk has come in then it is important to look for reasons why your baby is not lasting longer between feeds.

Only once a baby has regained his birth weight, and continues to have a steady weight gain, do I recommend that the times between feeds are extended, and only if the baby shows signs of happily going longer between feeds. By structuring your baby's feeds from early on, things should never get to a stage where he is having to cry to let you know he is hungry, as you will already be pre-empting his feeding needs.

From the very beginning it is important to differentiate between feeding, sleeping and social time. If you talk too much or overstimulate him while feeding, he could lose interest before taking a full feed, and then may not settle well to sleep, which could result in you feeding him to sleep, which, in the long term, can create sleep problems. Try to avoid talking on the telephone for long periods while feeding.

It is important, during the very early days, that you concentrate on the positioning of your baby on the breast to ensure that he feeds well. Do seek help from an experienced breast-feeding counsellor to make sure that you are getting the feeding position right. If you feed him in a rocking chair, do not be tempted to rock him while feeding, as he will think it is sleep time, and if he is sleepy while feeding, he will not feed so well and will need to feed again sooner. Sleepy babies are also often more prone to possetting back some of their feed. The aim of the CLB feeding routines is to ensure that when your baby is ready to increase milk feeds, you structure this increase into his daytime feeds to work with his daytime sleep. This will mean that, as soon as your baby is physically and mentally capable, he will sleep his longest spell in the night and not during the day.

Sleeping

It is essential for your baby's mental and physical development that he gets enough sleep; without the right amount he will become irritable, then fretful and inconsolable. A baby who is constantly tired will not feed efficiently, and therefore not sleep properly. As I have already mentioned, one of the most important things that you should try to remember in the early days is that very young babies can only stay awake for up to two hours before becoming tired. If your baby stays awake for longer than two hours he could become so exhausted that he will need a much longer sleep at his next nap time. This will have a knock-on effect, altering the rest of his routine, resulting in poor evening and night-time sleep. Therefore, it is essential that you structure the two-hourly awake period properly, so that the feeding and sleeping plan works well. In the early days some babies can only stay awake for an hour after a feed; this is fairly normal for babies who need more sleep. To determine whether your baby is a sleepy baby or not, look at his night-time sleep. If he can only stay awake for an hour at a time during the day, but settles well in the evening, and feeds and settles quickly during the night, he is a baby who needs more sleep. He will eventually manage to stay awake for longer amounts of time, provided you ensure that he is given the opportunity. You can do this by trying whenever possible to settle him in a quiet room for naps and, during his waking time, by having him in a bright, social and noisier environment. Create the contrast between naps and social time to help him learn when it's time to sleep and when it's time to play.

However, if he can only stay awake for an hour at a time during the day, but for longer spells during the night, it is possible that he has got his day and night muddled up, and it is worthwhile encouraging him to stay awake more during the day. Babies learn by association. It is very important that from day one he learns the right associations, and to differentiate between feeding, playing, cuddling and sleeping.

You will also find that there are some times of the day when your baby will stay awake for two hours quite happily, and other times when he will be tired after an hour. This is perfectly normal in the early days, which is why I say that babies can stay awake for up to two hours – not that they must stay awake for two hours. Along with the routines, the following guidelines will help your baby develop healthy sleeping habits:

- Try to keep him awake for a short spell after his day feeds.

- Do not let him sleep too long in the late afternoon.

- Do not feed him after 3.15pm, as it will put him off his next feed.

- Follow the same routine every evening; do not allow visitors around the baby during wind-down time and the bedtime routine.

- Do not let him get overtired; allow at least one hour for the bath, feed and wind-down time.

- Do not overstimulate him or play with him after his bath.

- Do not rock him to sleep in your arms; try to settle him in his cot before he goes into a deep sleep.

- If you use a dummy to wind him down, remove it before you put him in his cot.

- If he falls asleep on the breast or bottle, arouse him slightly before settling him in his cot.

Playing

All babies love to be cuddled, and talked and sung to. Research also shows that even very small babies like to look at simple books and interesting toys. For your baby to enjoy these things, it is important that you do them at the right time. The best time is usually approximately one hour after he is awake and has been fed. He should never be played with or overstimulated 20 minutes prior to his nap. Try to imagine how you would feel if you were just drifting off to sleep and someone came into the room and wanted to laugh and joke with you. I doubt you would be too happy about it, so try to respect that your baby needs the same quiet time before he goes off to sleep.

Pay particular attention to which toys you get your baby used to in his cot. Remember all toys and mobiles should be removed before sleep time. I find it a great help to divide toys and books into wake-up and wind-down ones. Musical cot mobiles and colourful baby gyms, plus black and white cloth cot books are all excellent for keeping young babies interested for short spells, during social time, as are postcards and posters that show single objects or faces. Use these toys only at social times and two or three different, less-stimulating toys for wind-down times.

Babies have very short concentration spans; constantly talking and handling a baby during the social time can often result in him becoming overstimulated. It's important to take the cue from your baby as to how much stimulation he can handle. Even from a very young age, babies should be encouraged to occupy themselves for short periods and have freedom to move. This is much more likely to happen if the baby is allowed to lie on his play mat or under his cot mobile, as he will be able to kick and move around more than when he is being held.

Cuddling

Babies need lots of cuddling, but it should always be done when your baby needs it, not when you need it. A baby needs energy to grow, so it is important that you do not overhandle his small body and exhaust him. While all babies need to be nurtured, they are not toys. Differentiate the type of cuddle during his play time from that of wind-down time. Wind-down cuddling should be about closeness of bodies. It is important that your baby is not cuddled to sleep while feeding. After one hour of being awake and fed he should be happy to spend a little time amusing himself; if you constantly cuddle him during play time, he will be less likely to respond to the cuddles that would normally help settle him for his nap. When cuddling him during the wind-down time, do not talk and avoid eye contact, as it can overstimulate him and result in him becoming overtired and not settling. Instead, just enjoy that peaceful connection and closeness that you feel with him.

Structuring the milk feeds during the first year

During the first few weeks, regardless of whether babies are breast- or formula-fed, very few can manage a strict four-hourly feeding pattern, and the aim of the CLB feeding routines is to ensure that the individual needs of all babies can be met. That is why I recommend that babies are fed three-hourly in the early days, and only when they have regained their birth weight and are gaining weight steadily should they be left to go longer for feeds (see page 184). By two weeks, if your baby has regained his birth weight and weighs over 3.2kg (7lb), he should manage to last 3–4 hours between some feeds, provided he is getting a full feed at the times stated in the routines. By structuring feeds in the early days you can achieve several slots of three-hour feeding and some of a four-hour stretch. If you structure his feeds according to the routines, the four-hour stretch between feeds should always happen between 10am–2pm and 7pm–7am. This would mean that a baby who fed at 6pm should get to 10pm, then feed again around 2–3am, then get to 5–7am.

Remember that the three-hour stretch between feeds is timed from the beginning of one feed to the beginning of the next; a baby starting to feed at 7am would then need to start his next feed at 10am. However, if you feel your baby is genuinely hungry before his next feed is due, as I have mentioned earlier, he must be fed – but it is also advisable to get to the root of the problem as to why he is not taking a full feed at the times stated in the routines. If you are breast-feeding, it may be that he needs longer on the second breast; if you are bottle-feeding, it may be that he needs an extra ounce at some feeds.

Between the second and fourth week, most babies who are gaining weight steadily (see page 184) are able to last slightly longer after one feed – usually four and a half to five hours. If you structure your baby's feeds, this will automatically be at the right time, i.e. between 11pm and 7am.

If your baby has been demand-fed and you are attempting to put him into a routine, I would advise that you look at the early routines and put him into a routine that seems nearest to his demand-fed pattern. For example, a nine-week-old baby may need to start on the two- to four-week schedule. When he is happy in that routine, you should be able to work your way through the next two sets of routines within 7–10 days. By the time he reaches 12 weeks, he should be happily feeding at the times stated in the routine for his age. However, although it may take slightly longer for him to sleep through the night, the important thing is that he is only feeding once in the night and gradually increasing the length of time he sleeps from his last feed, over a period of several weeks. Once the baby starts to sleep longer in the night, it is important to keep a close eye on how you structure feeds, as things can go wrong, particularly if you have been *too* strict. Remember the whole key to the CLB feeding routines is that they are flexible and that no baby should ever be forced to go longer before feeding than he is physically capable of. The following extract is from the diary of a mother with a five-week-old baby going approximately four hours between feeds. It shows how quickly things can go wrong, when a strict four-hourly routine is followed.

Tues	3am	7am	11am	3pm	7pm	11pm
Wed	3am	7am	11am	3pm	7pm	11pm
Thurs	4am	8am	12pm	4pm	8pm	12am
Fri	5am	9am	1pm	5pm	9pm	11pm
Sat	2am	6am	10am	2pm	6pm	10pm
Sun	2am	6am	10am	2pm	6pm	10pm

Aware that the feeding pattern was going haywire, the mother tried to get it back on track on the Friday night by waking the baby up at 11pm. This did not work, as the baby had taken a full feed at 9pm and was not hungry. It resulted in such a poor feed that the baby woke up at 2am needing a full feed, which meant a total backtrack on night feeding. Even if the mother had managed to settle the baby at 9pm with a smaller feed, it is unlikely the baby would have fed any better. The baby had only been asleep for one hour so it would have been very difficult to wake him up enough to feed properly.

As I mentioned earlier, the easiest way to keep your baby on track is to wake him at 7am. Once he is sleeping to 5am or 6am, he should be offered a top-up feed between 7am and 8am. This method will not only keep the rest of your feeds on track, but ensure that your baby's sleeping is kept on track as well and that he is ready to go to bed at 7pm.

The following advice will also ensure that your baby sleeps through the night as soon as he is physically able, and prepare him for the introduction of solids and the eventual reduction of milk feeds.

Understanding the routines for feeding

The 6–7am feed

- Depending on what time he fed in the night, your baby will probably wake up between 6am and 7am, but he should always be woken at 7am regardless. Remember that one of the main keys to getting your baby to sleep through the night is to ensure that once he is physically capable of bigger feeds, he takes his daily requirements between 7am and 11pm.

- Regardless of whether he is breast- or bottle-fed, the best way to keep a baby in a good routine is to begin the day at 7am.

Once he is sleeping through the night, he should be at his hungriest at this feed.

- During growth spurts, breast-fed babies should be given longer on the breast to ensure that their increased needs are met. If you have been expressing you can reduce this by 30ml (1oz) to ensure that his needs are immediately met. If you have not expressed, you can still follow the feeding times from the routine for your baby's age, but you will have to top him up with a short breast-feed before his daytime naps. If you do this for a week or so, this should help increase your milk supply. A sign that this has happened is that your baby will sleep well at the naps, and not be so interested in the next feed. Once this happens you can gradually decrease the length of time that you top-up for, until you are back on your original feeding schedule. A formula-fed baby should have his feeds increased by 30ml (1oz) when he is regularly draining his bottle.

- Once a baby starts to sleep longer in the night and is feeding between 5am and 6am, you may find that he will only take a small top-up feed between 7am and 8am, and then is hungrier much earlier for his next feed. When this happens you may find that until he sleeps right through to 7am, you will have to bring the 10.30–11am feed nearer to 10am and then offer a small top-up feed just prior to the lunchtime nap, to ensure that he sleeps well.

By seven months

- If your baby is eating a full breakfast of cereal, fruit and perhaps small pieces of toast, you should aim to cut back the amount offered to him from the breast or bottle. Try to divide the milk between a drink and with the cereal. Always try to encourage him to take at least 150–180ml (5–6oz) before he is given his solids.

- If you are breast-feeding, offer the first breast, then give him his solids and, finally, offer the second breast. Keep a very close watch that you do not allow him to increase his solids so much that he cuts back too much on his breast-feed.

- If your baby is still feeding in the night at this age it is important that you count any milk feeds after midnight as his breakfast milk. For example, if you give him a milk feed at 5am and then at 7am, you could find that he will be fussy with solids. Therefore I recommend that if he has been fed around 5–6am or earlier, go straight onto solids at around 7.30am, and then offer a small top-up milk feed after the solids.

- Your baby still needs a minimum of 600ml (20oz) a day, inclusive of milk used in cooking or on cereal.

- At this stage it is important your baby has a full breast-feed or 240 ml (8oz) of formula after bathing.

By ten months

- If your baby is formula-fed, try to encourage him to take all his milk from a beaker. Ensure that you still offer milk at the start of the meal. Once he has taken 150–180ml (5–6oz) of his milk, offer him some cereal. Then offer him the remainder of his milk again.

- It is important that he has at least 180–240 ml (6–8oz) of milk divided between the beaker and the breakfast cereal.

- If you are still breast-feeding, offer him first the breast then the solids, then offer him the breast again.

- Your baby needs a minimum of 500ml (18oz) a day, inclusive of milk used in cooking or on cereal, divided between two or three milk feeds.

The 10–11am feed

- During the first few weeks, the majority of babies who have fed between 6am and 7am will wake looking for a feed around 10am. Even if your baby does not do this it is important that you wake him. Remember that the aim is to ensure that your baby feeds regularly during the day so that he only needs to wake once for a feed between 11pm and 6–7am.

- Around six weeks, your baby may show signs of being happy to go longer from the 7am feed, and the 10am feed can gradually be pushed to 10.30am. However, a baby who is feeding at 5am or 6am and being topped up at 7.30–8am would probably still need to feed at 10am, as would the baby who has too small a feed at 7am. When this happens, it's best to offer a top-up feed prior to the lunchtime nap.

- Once he is sleeping through the night, or taking only a small feed in the night, he should have the biggest feed of the day at 6–7am. If he feeds well, he should be happy to last until 11am before needing another feed. However, if you feed him before he really needs it, he may not feed well and, as a result, may sleep poorly at the lunchtime nap. This will have a knock-on effect so that each subsequent feed and nap has to be given earlier and may result in the baby waking up at 6am or earlier the following morning.

- If you find that your baby can't wait until 10.30–11am for his feed, it is fine to feed him earlier. However I would recommend that you offer a top-up prior to the lunchtime nap to ensure that he does not wake up earlier because he was fed earlier.

- This feed would be the next one to be increased during growth spurts.

By six to seven months

- When your baby is eating breakfast, you can start to make this feed later, eventually settling somewhere between 11.30am and 12 noon. This will be the pattern for three meals a day at the end of six months, at which stage the milk feed will be replaced with a drink of water from a beaker.

- It is important that you introduce the tier system of feeding so that he gradually cuts back on the milk feed and increases his solids. As the weaning progresses, reduce the milk he has before solids and keep increasing the solids, but still offer milk after the solids.

- Some babies simply refuse to cut back on this milk feed. If you find that your baby is one, please refer to page 319 for suggestions on how to deal with this.

By seven months

- When your baby is on a proper balanced diet of solids, which includes protein with lunch, it is important that this feed should be replaced with a drink of water. If you find that your baby starts to wake up earlier from his lunchtime nap when the milk is stopped, then continue to offer him a small milk feed for a few more weeks prior to his lunch-time nap. If you do offer him a feed at this time you will find that he will probably cut down on his 2.30pm milk feed. This is not a problem, it just may mean that you have to bring his tea time solids forward to 4.45pm. It is better to do this than give a larger feed after 3pm and then he refuses solids or reduces the amount he is eating.

- Give the baby most of his solids before his drink so he doesn't fill up with liquid first.

The 2.30pm feed

- During the first few months, make this feed smaller so that your baby feeds really well at the 5–6.15pm feed, the exception being if your baby doesn't sleep well at lunchtime and needs feeding earlier with a top-up at 2.30pm. If, for some reason, the baby feeds badly at the 10am feed or was fed earlier, increase this feed accordingly so that he maintains his daily milk quota.

- If your baby is very hungry and regularly drains the bottle at this feed then you can give him a little extra, provided he does not take less at the next feed.

- For breast-fed babies, allow longer on the breast if he is not managing to get through happily to the next feed.

By eight months

- When your baby is having three full solid meals a day and his lunchtime milk feed has been replaced with water, you will probably need to increase this feed so that he is getting the daily milk quota he needs in three milk feeds.

- However, if he cuts back on the last milk feed of the day, it would be advisable to keep this milk feed smaller and make up the daily quota by using milk in cereals and cooking.

- Your baby still needs a minimum of 500–600ml (18–20oz) a day, inclusive of milk used in cooking and on cereal.

By nine to twelve months

- Bottle-fed babies should be given their milk from a beaker at this stage, which should automatically result in a decrease in the amount they drink.

- If this is not the case and your baby starts to lose interest in his morning or evening feed, you could cut right back on this feed. If he is getting 500–600ml (18–20oz) of milk a day (inclusive of milk used in cooking and on cereal), plus a full balanced diet of solids, you could cut this feed altogether.

- By one year of age your baby needs a minimum of 350ml (12oz) a day, inclusive of milk used in cooking and on cereal.

The 6–7pm feed

- It is important that your baby always has a good feed at this time if you want him to settle well between 7pm and 10pm.

- Try not to feed milk after 3.15pm, as it could put him off taking a really good feed at bedtime.

- In the first few weeks, this feed is split between 5pm and 6.15pm so that the baby does not get too frantic during his bath. Once your baby has slept through the night for two weeks, the 5pm feed can be dropped. I would not recommend dropping the split feed until this happens, as a larger feed at 6.15pm could result in your baby taking even less at the late feed, resulting in an earlier waking time. With many of the babies that I cared for, I kept giving them a split feed until solids were introduced to ensure that they were getting enough milk during the day. Once you eliminate the 5pm feed and your baby is taking a full feed after the bath, he could cut down dramatically on his late feed, which could result in an early waking.

- Breast-fed babies not settling at 7pm should be offered a top-up of expressed milk. Your milk supply may well be low at this time of the day.

By four to five months

- If your baby has started solids early, he should be given most of his milk before his solids, as milk is still the most important form of nutrition at this age.

- Most babies would be taking a full breast- or formula-feed at this age. At the 11am feed, give most of his milk feed first followed by the solids, then offer more milk at the end. As the weaning progresses you should gradually reduce the amount of milk he has before his solids and keep increasing the solids, but still offer milk at the end of the solids. In *The Contented Little Baby Book of Weaning*, there is a two-month weaning chart that gives day-to-day details on how gradually to increase solids and decrease the milk.

- For solids in the evening, I would recommend giving a small milk feed at 5pm, followed by the solids at 5.30pm. You can then delay his bath to around 6.25pm. After the bath he can then be offered the remainder of his milk feed. If formula feeding, it is advisable to make up two separate bottles to ensure that the milk is fresh.

- A breast-fed baby who has reached five months, is being weaned and is now starting to wake up before 10.30pm may not be getting enough milk at the bedtime feed. Try giving a top-up of expressed milk or formula after the bath. A baby who is not weaned would more than likely need to continue to have a split milk feed at 5–6.15pm until solids are introduced, and still be offered a late feed.

By six to seven months

- Most babies will now be having tea at 5pm followed by a full breast-feed or a full formula-feed after the bath. Once solids are established and the late feed is dropped, you may find that if you are breast-feeding, your baby starts to wake earlier. I would suggest that if this happens you should offer a top-up of expressed milk after the bedtime feed to ensure that he settles well at 7pm and sleeps through until the morning.

By ten to twelve months

- Bottle-fed babies should be taking all of their milk from a beaker at one year. Babies who continue to feed from a bottle after this age continue to take large amounts, which takes the edge off their appetite for solids. This can lead to fussiness with solids.

- Start encouraging your baby to take some of his daytime milk from a beaker at 10 months, so that by one year he is happy to take all of his bedtime feed from a beaker.

The late feed

- I strongly advise that parents of breast-fed babies should introduce bottles of either expressed milk or formula at this feed, no later than the second week. This will help share the feeding responsibilities with a partner or other carer.

- This also helps to avoid the common problem of a baby refusing to take a bottle at a later stage.

- A totally breast-fed baby under three months who continues to wake up between 2–3am may not be getting enough milk at the late feed, and can be offered a top-up of expressed or formula milk.

- If you choose to top up with expressed milk or formula rather than completely replacing the feed with a full bottle-feed, it is essential that you ensure that your baby has completely emptied the breast before he is offered the top-up feed.

- It is easier to tell whether formula-fed babies are getting enough milk at this feed. If you always increase the day feeds during your baby's growth spurts, he will probably never require more than 180ml (6oz) at this feed. However, some babies who weighed more than 4.5kg (10lb) at birth may reach a stage where they need more than this, until they are well established on solids.

- Refer to page 73 for calculating how much formula your baby needs each day, then see the example on page 75 for how to structure the feeds.

By three to four months

- If your baby has slept through the night until 7am for at least two weeks, then you can bring this feed forward by 10 minutes every three nights, until your baby is feeding at 10pm.

- If your baby is totally breast-fed and is still waking up early in the night, despite being topped up with expressed milk at the late feed, it may be worthwhile talking to your health visitor about replacing the late breast-feed with a formula-feed. Formula milk takes longer to digest and may help your baby to sleep longer in the night, although this is not guaranteed so think carefully about whether you mind introducing formula. Most formula-fed babies will be taking 210–240ml (7–8oz) a feed four or five times a day.

- If a formula-fed baby is not sleeping through the night at this age, it may be because he needs a little extra at this feed, and even if it means he cuts back on his morning feed, it may be worthwhile offering him an extra ounce or two. If he does cut down on the morning feed, you may find that for a short spell you need to bring the 11am feed forward to 10am and top him up with a small feed just prior to the lunchtime nap.

- Some babies simply start to refuse this feed at 3–4 months. However, if he goes through a growth spurt you may find that he starts to wake between 4–5am and will not settle back to sleep within 10 minutes or so, you would have to assume that it could be hunger and feed him.

- You can try to reintroduce the late feed again, perhaps doing a 'dream feed' around 11.30pm, but if your baby simply will not take a late feed, then you will have to accept that he may need feeding once in the night between midnight and 7am until he is well-established on solids.

- If your baby is waking twice in the night (i.e. 2am and 5am) or is not sleeping past 5am, you can try doing a split feed. Wake the baby at 9.45pm for this feed. Ensure he is wide awake either by changing his nappy, or by letting him have a kick around on his mat. Turn all the lights on. He should be feeding by 10pm. Try then to keep him up until 11pm by changing him or playing (whichever you didn't do at 9.45pm). Top him up just before he goes down at 11pm. By ensuring he is awake for longer at this feed and splitting it, he should only wake once in the night. Once this is established and he is going for a longer spell at night, you can slowly move the whole of this feed back to 10–10.30pm.

By four to eight months

- The majority of babies should be capable of sleeping through the night from their late feed at this age, provided they are having their daily intake of milk between 6–7am and 11pm.

- Some babies who are being exclusively breast-fed may only manage to get through to around 5am until they are weaned.

- Once your baby has been weaned and is established on three solid meals a day, the late feed should gradually reduce automatically. A baby who did not start solids until the recommended age of six months may still need this feed until he reaches seven months. By this time, provided the baby is taking enough milk and solids during the day, you should be able to gradually reduce the amount he takes and then eliminate it altogether.

The night feeds

- Newborn babies need to feed little and often during the first couple of weeks so when they wake it is best to assume that they are hungry and feed them.

- A newborn baby should never be allowed to go longer than three hours between feeds during the day and four hours between feeds in the night. This time is counted from the beginning of one feed to the beginning of the next.

- Once your baby has regained his birth weight, and weighs over 3.2kg (7lb) he should start to settle into the two- to four-week routine. Provided he feeds well between 10pm and 11pm, he should manage to sleep to nearer 2am.

By four to six weeks

- Most babies gaining the right amount of weight each week are capable of lasting a longer stretch between feeds during the night, as long as:

(a) The baby is taking his daily allowance of milk in the five feeds between 7am and 11pm.

(b) The baby is not sleeping more than four and a half hours between 7am and 7pm.

By six to eight weeks

- If your baby is gaining the right amount of weight each week but is still waking between 2am and 3am, despite taking a good feed at the late feed, it would be advisable to refer to Chapter 16 to check for possible reasons why he is not going longer in the night. It is worthwhile trying the core night method (see page 322).

- If the core night method does work, he will probably wake up again around 5am, at which time you can give him a full feed, followed by a top-up at 7–8am. This will help keep him on track with his feeding and sleeping pattern for the rest of the day.

- Within a week, babies usually sleep until nearer 5am, gradually increasing their sleep time until 7am. During this stage, when your baby is taking a top-up at 7–8am instead of a full feed, he may not manage to get through to 10.45–11am for his next feed. You may need to give him half his feed at 10am followed by the remainder at 10.45–11am, followed by a top-up just before he goes down for his lunchtime nap, to ensure that he does not wake up early from the nap.

- The other option is to feed your baby at 11.30pm and if this helps him to sleep a little longer in the night, do it for several nights, then gradually bring his feed back to the normal time and hopefully he will continue to sleep longer.

By three to four months

- Both breast-fed and bottle-fed babies should be able to go for one long spell during the night by this age, provided they are getting their daily intake of milk between 6–7am and 10–11pm.

- Your baby should be sleeping no more than three hours between 7am and 7pm. If your baby simply cannot cope on only three hours sleep during the day, you may have to accept that until his daytime sleep is reduced he may continue to wake up before 7am and need to be fed.

- Some breast-fed babies may still genuinely need to feed in the night if they are not getting enough at their late feed. If you are not already doing so, it is worth considering a top-up feed of expressed milk or formula, or a replacement formula feed at the late feed.

- Whether you are breast-feeding or bottle-feeding, if your baby's weight gain is good, and you are convinced he is waking up from habit, try leaving it for 15–20 minutes before going to him. Some babies will grumble on and off then settle themselves back to sleep.

- A baby of this age may still be waking up in the night because he is getting out of his covers. Tuck him in using the method described on page 6, or you can check out the video clip on contentedbaby.com

By four to five months

If your baby reaches five months and is still waking in the night, you probably need to persevere with his routine, paying increased attention to the timings of the feeds and the amount of daytime sleep he is getting. Try not to lose heart; some babies do need to feed in the night slightly longer. The most important thing is that he feeds and settles quickly and gets nearer to waking at 7am. Be reassured that he will very soon start to sleep through the night, provided you keep being vigilant with sleep times and feeding amounts. If you feel that he is showing signs that he is ready to be weaned, consult your health visitor or GP for advice as to whether he should begin earlier than the recommended six months (see Chapter 15 for more details).

The below chart shows which milk feeds are dropped first. By the time they reach one year most babies will be on only three milk feeds a day and some may have also cut out the mid-afternoon feed. Remember that the chart is only a guideline and within the routines there are details on how to adjust feeds.

Milk feeding chart for the first year

Age	Times
2–4 weeks	2–3am, 7am, 10am, 11–11.15am, 2–2.30pm, 5pm, 6–6.15pm, 10–10.30pm
4–6 weeks	3–4am, 7am, 10.30am, 2–2.30pm, 5pm, 6–6.15pm, 10–10.30pm

6–8 weeks	4–5am, 7am, 10.45am, 2–2.30pm, 5pm, 6.15pm, 10–10.30pm
8–12 weeks	5–6am, 7am, 10.45–11am, 2–2.15pm, 5pm, 6.15pm, 10–10.30pm
3–4 months	7am, 11am, 2.15–2.30pm, 5pm, 6–6.15pm, 10–10.30pm
4–6 months	7am, 11am, 2–2.30pm, 5pm, 6.15–6.30pm, 10pm
6–9 months	7am, 2.30pm, 6.30pm
9–12 months	7am, 2.30pm, 6.30–7pm

Structuring daytime sleep during the first year

The whole aim of the CLB routines is to ensure that the timings of feeds fit in with your baby's daily sleep requirements. A baby who does not feed well during the day will not sleep well during the day; and to ensure good night-time sleep for your baby it is essential that you structure his daytime sleep. Too much can result in night-time wakings. Too little can result in an overtired, irritable baby who has difficulty settling himself to sleep, and who falls asleep only when he is totally exhausted.

When following the routines it is important to remember that they are simply guidelines to help you decide just how long your baby can stay awake, before he needs to nap.

Of course, if you have a baby who is only staying awake an hour at a time during the day, and partying for several hours in the night, this is a different matter, and you may have to try harder to encourage him to stay awake longer during the day if excessive night-time waking is to be avoided. Please refer to page 104 for details on how to deal with this problem.

> ### Top Tip
>
> Most babies in the early days can stay awake happily for up to two hours before needing a nap. I am not saying that they *must* stay awake for the full two hours, only that it is important that they do not stay awake longer than two hours, if overtiredness is to be avoided. So, if during the early days, you find that your baby is only staying awake for an hour or an hour and a half at a time, you do not need to worry providing he is sleeping well at night; he is obviously a baby that needs more sleep.

The importance of nap times

Infant sleep expert Marc Weissbluth (see page 364) has carried out extensive research into the nap patterns of more than 200 children. He says that napping is one of the healthy habits that sets the stage for good overall sleep and explains that a nap offers the baby a break from stimuli and allows him to recharge for further activity. Charles Schaefer PhD, Professor of Psychology at Fairleigh Dickinson University in Teaneck, New Jersey, supports this and says: 'Naps structure the day, shape both the baby's and the mother's moods, and offer the only opportunity for Mom to relax or accomplish a few tasks.'

Several leading experts on child care are in agreement that naps are essential to a baby's brain development. John Herman PhD, infant sleep expert and Associate Professor of Psychology and Psychiatry at the University of Texas, says: 'If activities are being scheduled to the detriment of sleep, it's a mistake. Parents should come after sleeping and eating.' I couldn't agree more. By 3–4 months, most babies are capable of sleeping 11–12 hours at night (with a sleepy feed at 10pm), provided their daytime sleep is no more than three to three and a half hours, divided between two or three naps a day. If you want your baby to sleep from 7–7.30pm to 7–7.30am, it is very important you structure these naps so that he has his longest nap at midday, with two shorter ones in the morning and late afternoon. While it may be more convenient to let your baby have a longer nap in the morning followed by a shorter nap in the afternoon, this can lead to the following problem:

Once he reduces his daytime sleep naturally, he is most likely to cut back on his late-afternoon nap. His longest nap of the day would then be in the morning. By late afternoon he will be exhausted and need to go to bed by 6.30pm. This could result in him waking up at 6am. If you manage to get him to have a nap in the late afternoon, you could then be faced with the problem of him not settling well at 7–7.30pm.

Understanding the sleeping routine

If you want your baby to settle well in the evening and sleep his longer spell at night then you must work hard at establishing a good morning nap in the early days. I know how exhausting it can be when you have to get up in the night to feed your baby and how ridiculous it may sound that you should wake your baby at 7am in the morning, but the truth is that if you are prepared to put the effort in during the first few weeks and start your baby's day at 7am, then you stand a much better chance of your baby starting to sleep his long spell at night sooner than if you allow each day to begin at random times. Of course I am well aware that some babies will sleep their longer spell at night regardless of what time they wake in the morning, but believe me they are in the minority!

The first month

If you wake your baby at 7am and give him a good feed, he will more than likely manage to stay awake between one and one and a half hours before being ready to sleep again; he should then sleep until the next feed time at 10am. If you find that your baby is falling asleep at 8–8.30am and then waking up much earlier than 10am, then I would suggest that hunger is the problem and would recommend that you offer him a small top-up prior to his morning nap to ensure that he sleeps well until nearer 10am. Once you reach a stage where you are having to wake your baby up nearer 10am you can then gradually reduce the top-up feed and eventually eliminate it altogether.

By the end of the first month your baby should hopefully be managing to stay awake nearer 8.30am and then sleep until nearer 10am. This is based on him sleeping to nearer 7am. If your baby is not sleeping to 7am, then please refer to page 100 on how to deal with early morning waking. At this stage your baby may still be waking around 6am, and it is essential that you get him back to sleep as quickly as possible so that you can keep him on track with his feeding and sleeping during the rest of the day.

Four to eight weeks

Until a proper sleep pattern has been established, try to ensure that this nap takes place in a quiet room if possible. Once a proper daytime routine has been established, this nap could at times be taken in the pram if you have to go out, but do remember to try and be home by 9.45am so you can wake him up by 10am. By the time your baby reaches four weeks he should show signs of managing to stay awake longer and longer periods, with the aim of him staying awake by up to one and a half hours to two hours by the time he is eight weeks. Of

> ## Top Tip
>
> When establishing a routine it is essential that whatever happens with feeding and sleeping over the 24-hour day, you have a set time to start the day and a set time to end the day. Without this you will find that for many weeks and often months your baby's routine will change on a day-to-day basis.

course all babies are different, but encouraging your baby to stay awake for longer periods at this first waking time of the day will most certainly help his night-time sleep. If your baby is not showing signs of staying awake longer between 7am and 9am, then you need to look at two things: what time he is waking in the night and how much he is feeding at 7am. The main causes of a baby not staying awake longer from 7am are usually because:

- He is waking at 6am and not returning to sleep quickly. If this the case please refer to page 100 on how to ensure that your baby sleeps nearer to 7am.

- The 6am feed can result in a poor top-up feed between 7am and 8am. If your baby is feeding at 6am and refusing a top-up feed or only taking a very small one between 7am and 8am and not sleeping well at the morning nap, then you should try topping up 15 minutes prior to the time of the morning nap.

Eight to twelve weeks

By this stage most babies are managing to stay awake nearer two hours. However some babies who need more sleep will be ready to sleep before two hours is up. It is really important not to confuse a baby who needs more sleep with a baby whose body clock needs adjusting. A baby who needs more sleep will fall asleep earlier than 9am, then sleep through to nearer 10am or have to be woken, sleep well at the lunchtime nap, settle well by 7pm and then sleep a longer spell from the late feed.

If your baby reaches eight to twelve weeks and is sleeping to nearer 7am, but then falling asleep long before 9am and waking up after 30–40 minutes, he will then need to have his lunch time nap brought forward, which has a knock-on effect for the whole day. If you find this is happening, I would recommend that you try splitting the morning nap for a short spell so that he can then get through to nearer 12 noon for his lunch time nap (see page 137).

Three to six months

If your baby is sleeping well until nearer 7am, at this stage you should have managed to establish a morning nap of around 45 minutes from 9am. Occasionally I have had some babies who would cut back on their morning nap at this age and be awake from 9.30am. Some I could get to nearer 11.30am for their next sleep so that I could keep the lunchtime on track, but with those I couldn't I had to choose between putting them down around 11.15am or doing a split morning nap.

I usually always went for the split nap, which meant that I could get them to nearer 12/12.30pm for the lunchtime nap. I found that with babies of this age, unlike much younger babies, by putting them down around 11.15am meant they would be awake around 1.30–2pm, which would mean a split nap in the afternoon. I personally found it easier to do the split nap in

Splitting naps

Morning

If your baby wakes from his morning nap at 9.30am, try putting him down earlier for a cat-nap between 8.30–8.45am but only allow him 20–30 minutes. Then aim for another short cat-nap of 10–15 minutes between 10.30–11am. This should get him through to nearer 12–12.30pm for his lunchtime nap, when you can then follow the routine as normal.

Afternoon

If your baby wakes early from his lunchtime nap at 1.30–2pm and can't manage to get to 4.30pm for a late afternoon nap, let him have a short nap around 2.30–3pm of no more than 10–15 minutes, followed by a cat-nap between 4.30–5pm so that he will still be able to settle at 7pm.

The important thing to remember when doing split naps is not to exceed the daily sleep total.

the morning than in the afternoon, as most babies are harder to get to sleep late afternoon once they are past three months. Whichever way you choose to deal with a short morning nap, remember that this stage will not last forever and that between six and nine months most babies will automatically cut back on their morning nap themselves.

Six to nine months

If your baby continues to sleep well until nearer 7am at this stage you will probably notice that he is not falling to sleep quite so quickly at 9am. Even if he isn't showing signs of wanting to go down later I would actually encourage a later put down by gradually extending the time he is awake in the morning by a couple of minutes every few days, until he eventually goes down closer to 9.30am. This will enable you to push the lunchtime nap on to 12.30–2.30pm, which will in turn help you (if you have not already done so) eliminate the late afternoon altogether. If you do not reduce the morning nap you risk the problem of your baby cutting back on his lunchtime sleep, which will of course mean that you have keep offering a short late afternoon nap to get him through happily until bedtime. In my experience the majority of babies can start to fight sleep later in the day, which can result in the baby refusing to nap then having to be settled earlier for bed, which can result in early morning waking. Once early morning waking establishes itself it is then difficult to push the morning nap later, hence the importance of you always being one step ahead of your baby's needs and pre-empting when to make adjustments. Please refer to page 100 for advice and information on how to avoid early morning waking.

Nine to twelve months

While some babies will reduce the time of this nap even further and only sleep for 15–20 minutes or even cut it out altogether, others will continue to have a morning nap into the second year. You will know your baby is ready to drop this nap when he starts taking a long time to settle, and ends up sleeping only 10–15 minutes of his 30–45 minute nap. Other telling signs that this nap may need to be cut down or perhaps dropped is when a baby is waking up during his lunchtime nap, in the night or early morning, where he had previously slept well. If a baby is resisting sleep at his morning nap and for a couple of weeks manages to get through to his lunchtime nap happily, cut the morning nap out altogether.

It can be tricky going from two naps down to one, and getting rid of the morning nap often results in a baby's midday nap being brought forward too early. This earlier lunchtime nap obviously means an earlier wake-up time from the nap, which in turn results in the baby being so overtired when he is put to bed that he goes into a deep sleep very quickly, or being put to bed to early to avoid overtiredness. Both scenarios can result in early morning wakening and soon the baby gets into the habit of waking up early. He can then become so tired that rather than the parents being able to reduce and eliminate the morning nap, they find themselves having to increase it so their baby gets through happily to the lunchtime nap. What many parents do not realise is that during the transition period of dropping the morning nap, they may need to start the lunchtime nap later, thereby slightly reducing it, until the morning nap is totally eliminated. Once the morning nap has successfully been dropped, the lunchtime nap can then start and end at the usual time.

If your baby is over nine months and showing signs of waking earlier, not being ready for his morning nap, or reducing his lunchtime nap (all signs that a change in sleeping needs is imminent), I would suggest the following tips to help to prevent early morning waking becoming a problem.

Top Tips

- Gradually push the morning nap on from 9.30am so that your baby is going down nearer to 9.45–10am. Once they are happily going through to this time, gradually reduce the length of the nap to 15 minutes. You can then push the lunchtime nap on to nearer 12.45 pm and allow a nap of no more than two hours.

- If your baby is showing signs of not being ready to sleep at 9.45–10am, do not be tempted to drop the morning nap as doing it too early means that his lunchtime nap could come too soon, resulting in him going to bed in the evening either overtired or early.

- Keep pushing your baby's morning nap on until he manages to get close to 11am, then allow a nap of five to ten minutes. Once he is managing to get through to 12.45–1pm for his lunchtime nap with only this short nap, you should be able to cut it out altogether and get him through to around 12.15–12.30pm for his nap, which would then be increased to two hours.

- If you find that your baby is becoming too tired to eat a proper lunch, you can always bring his lunch forward slightly for a short period until his body clock adjusts to the new nap times. I usually find that once they have had lunch they perk up enough to get through to 12.15–12.30pm.

The important thing to remember if you want to avoid early morning waking is not to become complacent about your baby's sleeping habits. If you have enjoyed a really good routine for nearly a year, it is all too easy to assume that your baby is a naturally a good sleeper and that nothing will go wrong. Being one step ahead of your baby's sleeping needs by reading about the next stage and gradually reducing daytime sleep is the best way to avoid the dreaded early morning waking.

Lunchtime nap

This should always be the longest sleep of the day. By establishing a good lunchtime nap, you will ensure that your baby is not too tired to enjoy afternoon activities, and that bedtime is relaxed and happy. Recent research shows that a nap between noon and 2pm is deeper and more refreshing than a later nap because it coincides with the baby's natural dip in alertness.

A baby who goes to bed overtired is much more likely to wake up early in the morning, hence the importance of ensuring that he is not going too long from the time he wakes up from his afternoon nap to the time he goes to bed. During the first few months this is unlikely to happen as most babies will still be on three naps a day, but as they cut out the third nap of the day, if the lunchtime nap is a short one, then it most certainly could become a problem. Hence the reason for thinking ahead when establishing nap times for your baby.

The first month

Regardless of how long your baby has slept during the morning nap I would recommend that you wake him up no later than 10am so that you can keep his feeding and sleeping on track. As babies of this age can rarely stay awake much longer than one to one and half hours, you should aim for a lunchtime nap between 11.30am and 2pm, although some very sleepy babies may need to be settled by 11.15am. If, for some reason, his morning nap was much shorter, then you could allow him two and a half hours. In the early days, a lunchtime nap may sometimes go wrong and he make wake up earlier. When this happens I always recommend that you feed your baby, treating it like a night feed and try to get your baby back to sleep. If your baby doesn't settle back to sleep, he will not make it make it through to 4pm happily. I find the best way to deal with this is to allow a short cat-nap of 15–30 minutes after the 2–2.30pm feed, then a further 30 minutes at 4.30pm. This should stop him becoming overtired and irritable, and get things back on track so that he settles to sleep well at 7pm.

Four to eight weeks

Your baby should start to show signs of managing to stay awake a bit longer between feeds at this stage, and will hopefully manage to stay awake from 7am to nearer 9am. If your baby is sleeping a lot longer than one hour at the morning nap and not settling well at the lunchtime nap, or waking up after an hour at the lunchtime nap, despite being offered a top-up prior to the nap, the cause is probably too long a nap in the morning. When this happens the afternoon often ends up with a series of cat-naps with the baby often becoming very irritable. In these circumstances I would recommend that you reduce the amount of sleep your baby is having at the morning nap for a couple of weeks by doing a split morning nap of 30 minutes and 15 minutes (see split naps page 137). This will see his morning sleep reduced by around 30–45 minutes, which should help him sleep better at the lunchtime nap.

At this age, hunger is often the reason for the baby not sleeping so long at the lunchtime nap, therefore I would always recommend offering a top-up before the lunchtime nap to eliminate the possibility of hunger.

During the second month I would also recommend that you start to ensure your baby is going down sleepy but definitely awake and aware he is going into his bed.

Eight to twelve weeks

Between eight and twelve weeks you may find that your baby starts to wake up after 30–40 minutes of being settled to sleep and refuses to settle back to sleep. As before, I would recommend feeding your baby and trying to settle him back to sleep, but I think that you also have to look at whether he is going into his bed too sleepy. At this age it is really important that he learns to settle himself to sleep otherwise you will see a pattern of him only sleeping short spells of 30–40 minutes at a time, instead of one longer spell of two to two and half hours.

If your baby has been used to being fully swaddled and you find that he is not sleeping so well because he dislikes his arms being out, I would recommend that you compromise and semi-swaddle him. By tucking in only one arm to the swaddle it can help the baby adapt more easily to being un-swaddled.

Three to six months

If you have not already done so I would recommend that you gradually reduce the morning nap to no more than 45 minutes. Between three and six months your baby should be managing to stay awake near enough two hours at his waking times, which means that his lunchtime nap will be coming nearer to 12 noon. Sometimes babies who have been sleeping well at lunchtime will suddenly start to wake mid-way through their nap or much earlier than usual. If this happens between four and six months it could be genuine hunger and I would recommend that you go back to feeding your baby around 10.30am so that you can offer him a bigger top-up prior to his lunchtime nap.

Six months onwards

From around six months I would recommend that you gradually move the morning nap on from 9am to 9.30am which will enable you to move the lunchtime nap on to nearer 12.30pm. Once solids are introduced and your baby is on three meals a day with the 11am milk feed gradually reducing and being replaced with a full solid meal, you will want to aim for him to have his lunchtime solids nearer 12 noon so that there will be a big enough gap between breakfast and lunch for him to eat his solids well. If he is sleeping less than two hours at lunchtime, check that his morning nap between 7am and 12 noon is no more than 30 minutes. If he is taking longer to go to sleep and not falling asleep until around 9.45am, it is important to still wake him by 10am. Although not that common I have known some babies between six and twelve months who need to cut their morning nap down to around 15–20 minutes, in order to keep the long lunchtime nap. Please refer to page 139 on reducing or dropping the morning nap, if you think your baby is showing signs of needing to cut his.

Nine to twelve months

If your baby has difficulty in settling for the nap, or is waking up after one to one and a half hours, you might have to cut the morning nap back even further or get rid of it altogether.

Late-afternoon nap

This is the shortest nap of the three, and the one the baby should drop first. It is essential that your baby learns to sleep in places other than his bed as it also allows you the freedom to get out and about.

The first month

If your baby sleeps well at the lunchtime nap and wakes around 2–2.15pm, he will probably be ready to have a nap near 3.30–4pm. Some very sleepy babies may not manage to get to 3.30–4pm and fall asleep nearer 3/3.30pm. If this happens I would be inclined to let them have a short cat nap, then wake them up for a short spell and then let them have a further nap until 5pm. It is tempting to let them sleep right through to 5pm, but if you continue to do this, by the time they reach two or three weeks you would probably encounter evening settling problems because they had slept too much late afternoon.

Four to eight weeks

Once your baby is in his second month, provided he is sleeping well at lunchtime, he should manage to stay awake longer after the 2–2.30pm feed, getting nearer to 4.15pm before needing a nap. If he is still not managing to stay awake until nearer 4.15pm, then it would be advisable to encourage a couple of cat naps, totalling about one hour, rather than allowing him to sleep one hour solid. For example, if he falls asleep at 3.30pm and sleeps solidly until 4.30pm, he would then probably need to be in bed by 6.15pm if he was not to become overtired. If you allowed him to sleep solidly nearer to 5pm then, as already mentioned, you could find it difficult to settle him at 7pm because he will have had too much sleep late afternoon. Try to aim for no more than one hour of sleep between 2pm and 5pm, even if you have to split the naps (see page 137 for more information on split naps).

Eight to twelve weeks

Babies who are sleeping well at night and following the correct nap times for their age, will start to cut back on their late afternoon nap and should now manage to get to 4.30pm for this nap. Some babies will then cat nap on and off between 4pm and 5pm and others will actually start to stay awake longer and not fall asleep.

Three months onwards

Most babies who are sleeping well at their other two naps will gradually cut right back on this sleep until they are only having 10–15 minutes at the late afternoon nap. When this happens it is important that you try to push this nap nearer to 4.30–4.45pm. If they cut back the nap or have it earlier, then you risk the problem of them going down much earlier or becoming overtired and not settling well at bedtime. Even if your baby doesn't show signs of cutting his late afternoon nap back at this stage, I would recommend that you gradually encourage him to stay awake a couple of minutes longer every few days so that he eventually does drop it. I certainly found that babies who dropped their late afternoon nap by the time they were three to four months old were much more likely to sleep through the night sooner.

Obviously if your baby is not sleeping well at the lunchtime nap, then the late afternoon nap will have to stay in place until the lunchtime nap issues are resolved.

Adjusting the routines

Birth to six months

I have tried many different routines over the years and, without exception, I have found the 7am to 7pm routine to be the one in which tiny babies and young infants are happiest. It fits in with their natural sleep rhythms and their need to feed little and often. I urge parents to try to stick to the original routine whenever possible. Once your baby reaches the stage of only needing four feeds a day and needs less daytime sleep, it is possible to change the routine without affecting your baby's natural needs for the right amount of sleep and number of feeds.

Up to the age of six months, the following points should be noted when planning a routine:

- In the very early weeks, to avoid more than one waking in the night, you must fit in at least five feeds before midnight. This can only be done if your baby starts his day at 6am or 7am.

- An 8am to 8pm routine in the first few weeks would mean your baby would end up feeding twice between midnight and 7am. The other problem with an 8am to 8pm routine with a very young baby, is that regardless of doing a feed at midnight they nearly always wake between 6–7am, and need to be settled back to sleep.

Six months onwards

From six months, when your baby has started solids and you have dropped the late feed, it is easier to adjust the routine. If your baby has been sleeping regularly to 7am, it could be possible to change to a 7.30am or 8am start, and push the rest of the routine forward. Your baby would obviously need to go to sleep later in the evenings. If you want your baby to sleep later in the morning, try the following:

- Cut right back on the morning nap, so that your baby is ready to go to bed at 12–12.30pm.

- Allow a nap of no longer than two hours at lunchtime and no late afternoon nap.

Adjusting the routine for nursery

Babies can start at nursery at many different ages but the routines set out below are for babies of around six months old.

Sleeping

During the first few weeks, however well your baby sleeps at nursery, he may well be tired when he returns. The adjustments he needs to make, the new surroundings and people are a lot for him to take in. Although you are eager for him to remain with his usual bedtime, in the first weeks after starting nursery you may need to make this slightly earlier until he is more settled. As he may not be at nursery every day you can adjust bedtime depending on what has happened during the day. On the days he is at home and at weekends, you can remain on your present routine if it suits you. Once he has got used to being at nursery, he will probably manage to go back to his usual schedule, but with a slightly shorter lunchtime nap.

Some babies at nursery never manage to do the long lunchtime nap and only manage an hour or even less. This can be a problem in the very early days until they adapt to getting through the day on a shorter lunchtime nap. If this happens with your baby it may be that you have to tell the nursery to let him have a slightly longer morning nap, if he will. Then his lunchtime nap, although shorter, will come later but it will help him get through to bedtime without becoming so overtired. It may be that at nursery they have to follow the sleep pattern of the daytime sleep being split into two equal naps morning and afternoon, as opposed to one shorter morning nap and a longer lunchtime nap. On the days he is at home, there is no reason why you can't revert back to his normal routine and do the shorter nap in the morning and longer nap at lunchtime. I find that in time most babies will eventually adapt to a different routine at nursery to the one they have at home.

If your baby will not take a longer morning nap and ends up having two shorter naps, then another option is when you pick him up drive around an extra ten minutes, to see if he will take a short cat nap in the car. Although this can seem like a real inconvenience at a time when you just want to get your baby home, it is in my opinion worth it, if it helps your baby get through to bedtime without becoming overtired. Remember this will only last until your baby learns to adjust to shorter naps at nursery and manages to stay awake longer from the time he wakes up from his afternoon nap. The important thing to remember is not to exceed the total daytime sleep recommended for his age.

Feeding

Most nurseries do lunch around 11.30am and tea at 3.30pm, so if your baby has had a good lunch and tea at nursery, you can't expect your baby to eat another full meal when he gets home. However, you can't expect him to get through from 3.30–4pm to the morning without further solids. Therefore he will need to be offered a small snack when he gets home to get him through to bedtime happily but don't offer him so much food that he reduces his bedtime milk feed. Some nurseries are prepared to offer babies a snack instead of a full tea at 3pm; it is worth checking with your nursery if they are happy to do this for the first few weeks at least. If not then you will need to balance out the solids he has at nursery with the solids he has when you get him home. As you still want him to take a good milk feed, I would recommend that you offer solids no later than 5.45pm and not so much of them that it puts him off his bedtime milk, which is still important at this age. As he will be quite tired and time is limited, I would recommend quick meals: a small bowl of pasta with sauce, a thick vegetable soup with bread, small pizza slices or mini sandwiches are all quick and easy options. For babies who are very tired and fussy at this time I used to find that a bowl of cereal would sometimes do the trick.

Adjusting the routine for daytime outings

It is so important for both you and your baby to get out in the fresh air, to meet friends or visit places that are stimulating and fun. Seeing friends and family can be a lifeline in the early days when you are making that challenging adjustment to parenthood. My routines are intended to help you enjoy your contented babies and find freedom, not hinder it. The following advice will help you learn how to adjust your baby's routines, without it being detrimental to his sleep.

Obviously I advise to stick to the routine as much as you can, but I do understand that it might be difficult when you have planned a day out. For short trips, such as a walk in the park or coffee with a friend, you can easily stick to the routine by simply arranging your outing around your baby's sleep time. Please note, however, that this does not work with very young babies, who usually fall asleep as soon as the pram starts moving. In the case of very young babies, I would suggest that an outing actually coincides with their sleep time, to avoid them sleeping for too long during the day.

For longer trips, you will have to change the routine slightly – but don't worry, this can be done without losing all the effort you have put in to establishing your baby's routine!

The following suggestions should help, but please remember that they are guidelines. You know your baby best, so if you have to make further adaptations, please do so.

Managing sleeping and naps when going out to lunch

If you have a baby or toddler who can easily sleep two hours in his pushchair during the lunchtime nap, I would definitely recommend you stick to that. The advantage of this is that you needn't change the routine too much, and your child can stick to his regular sleep and mealtimes. A lot of babies do not manage to stay asleep for longer than 45 minutes in their pushchair. If this is happens, you can try the following adjustments:

- As a one-off, let him sleep one and a half hours for his morning nap (should he want to sleep that long). This will keep him happy until after lunch, at which time you can let him have another 45–60 minutes in his buggy or in the car mid-afternoon. If your baby will not sleep longer than 30–40 minutes in the morning, don't worry – just accept that he may only sleep for 30–40 minutes at lunchtime and then wake up. Even if he is not due a feed, offer it to him anyway. The last thing you want is a wailing baby in a restaurant or at a friend's house, just because you are determined to stick to the routine! If he takes half his feed around 1pm, then give him a top-up at 2–2.30pm before letting him have a further nap in the buggy. He is unlikely to sleep longer than 45 minutes, so he will need a further short nap late afternoon. On a day out, remember it is not a catastrophe if he has to have three short naps of 30–45 minutes each.

- If you need to travel for an hour or so to get where you're going, then you can let your baby have his morning nap in the car. Try and leave home about 10 minutes before your baby normally goes down, to ensure he doesn't get over-tired or cranky in the car. He can then have his lunchtime nap in his travel cot. Depending on his age and whether he can stay awake well in the car, you can slightly reduce the lunchtime nap so that he can have a nap on the way home without it affecting the total amount of daily sleep he has had.

- If for some reason the plan goes wrong and he sleeps between 5–6pm, then don't worry – it just means he won't be ready to go down at 7pm. Just keep an eye on him for signs of tiredness and settle him around 7.30–8pm when he is sleepy. Start the following day as usual, even if he has gone down later.

Evening routine at a friend's house

If you are spending the whole day at a friend's house, it is a good idea to try and keep the evening routine similar to home. Explain to your friend what your baby's routine is, and ask if it would be ok to give your baby a bath there. This means your baby can drink his milk and get into the car at 7pm already in his sleep suit/pyjamas and sleeping bag for the journey home. If he is not overtired from the day's activities, he will probably enjoy having a bath somewhere different! Once at home, with luck you will be able to transfer your sleeping baby straight into his cot. If he doesn't settle, offer a top-up of milk. This may result in him taking less milk at breakfast, but don't worry as his milk intake will even out over the day once he is back in the normal routine.

If, for whatever reason, you are unable to give your baby a bath, don't worry. Just ensure that he has a good wash the next morning!

Fresh air and exercise

Wherever you may be on your day out, do try and let your baby get some fresh air and exercise. If you are going to a friend's house or visiting family for the whole day, it should still be possible for a baby to have a little kick on a play mat. It is also important to get the baby out for a stroll in the fresh air. Fresh air usually helps babies to sleep better, so even if your baby sleeps in the car, as long as he has had lots of fresh air and some exercise, he should still settle well by bedtime. When out with a very young baby, try and avoid passing him round too much so he doesn't end up being in someone's arms most of the time. I am sure family and friends will want a cuddle, but also explain how much your baby likes his little kick!

The next day ...

Some babies are naturally more sociable, while others find busy social activities overwhelming. The latter baby might be more tired after a day out than a more socially comfortable baby. If your baby seems exhausted after a busy day, make sure the next one is peaceful and predictable to restore their sense of security and avoid them becoming overtired. Let your baby guide you on this. Remember that a quiet day at home and a walk in the park might seem boring to you, but it can be a great source of comfort to a baby who needs routine in which to develop social skills at their own pace.

Top Tip

The important thing to remember when you are planning days away is not to fret if your baby's routine slips a little. I have always found that when a baby is contented, he is also adaptable.

Adjusting the routine for evenings out

I realise the thought of taking your baby out in the evening might seem very daunting, especially if you have worked hard to get him into a good routine, but having worked in the Far East, Middle East and Italy where it was common for babies to be taken to family gatherings in the evening, I know from personal experience that it is possible to adapt the routines when necessary. Also, the earlier that you learn to do this, the more confident you will become about accepting occasional evening invitations.

As a new parent you need the support of your family and friends. In order to strengthen and build these relationships, it is important that you don't foster resentment as others may not initially understand your concern for your baby's routine, and will feel neglected if you turn down all their invitations. The key thing is compromise. Although there will be times when you do decide to turn down an appealing invitation, there will be others when you decide it is more important to attend than to ensure your baby is put in his cot at 7pm.

Depending on the age of your baby, there are two ways to approach the possibility of taking your baby along with you to a party. If your baby is over six months and in a well-established routine, ask your hosts if you may arrive early to carry out your baby's bed- and bath-time routine at their home. In this way, you will be able to settle the baby in a travel cot in a bedroom upstairs before the other guests arrive. However, if for any reason your baby does not settle as usual – perhaps because he senses that he is not in his usual environment – don't worry or become anxious. Accept the situation as it is and follow the advice below for younger babies.

If it is not an option to carry out your evening routine at the venue, when, for example, going to a restaurant, it is still possible for you to accept the invitation, as long as you acknowledge and understand that for this one evening your baby's routine will have to be altered, as outlined below. In this instance, the key thing to remember is that for the duration of the party, you treat your baby's feeds and sleeps as daytime ones, rather than as evening or night ones, and you don't carry out your usual bed- and bath-time routine.

By following my guidelines, I hope you will begin to have the confidence to accept invitations and learn how to adapt the routines, safe in the knowledge that your baby can come too, and will continue to be a contented little baby – and you will be a contented, relaxed parent!

Guidelines for successful socialising with contented babies

- During the afternoon of the event, try to take your baby out for a walk. I have always found that fresh air helps to settle babies – and it will energise you, ready for the night ahead.

- If your baby is on solids, feed him his tea as usual – or slightly earlier in order to give yourself time to get ready.

- Before you leave for the party, offer him what would normally be his bedtime feed, but treat it like a daytime feed. It is important that you do not send out signals that it is time for bed.

- Remember to pack a spare set of clothes, blanket, some favourite toys and, if you are formula-feeding, everything you will need for two milk feeds.

- Once at the venue, your friends will be keen to say hello to your new baby. Try to keep him in his buggy or car seat, which will avoid him being passed around and too many people cuddling him. Explain that normally he is asleep at this time, and that you want to avoid him becoming overstimulated which could result in him getting very upset, and you having to leave the party early.

- If your baby had a short sleep in the car he will probably get a second wind and be happy to stay awake for one to two hours before he needs to sleep again. If he did not sleep in the car it is important that you keep an eye on him so that you can encourage him to nap before he gets overtired. You may have to offer him a small top-up feed to get him to sleep. Try to find a quiet spot where you can do this. After his feed, settle him in his buggy, in a quiet corner of the party, tucking him in with blankets as you would do in his cot.

- As your baby may sense that he is not in his normal surroundings, you may need to jiggle the buggy a little to help him settle and go to sleep. With your baby asleep, choose one or two trusted friends who will take turns on 'buggy patrol' with you and your partner, every fifteen minutes. This way you will be able to mingle and chat without worrying about your baby all the time.

- Be realistic about how long your baby will sleep for. If he sleeps soundly for two or three hours that is great, but he may only sleep for 30–40 minutes. In this case, you can try to settle him back by gently jiggling the buggy. If this doesn't work, treat the sleep like you would a short daytime nap, and accept that he may be awake for another hour or two. If he is irritable you may have to offer him another small feed and some cuddles.

Once back home, how you deal with settling him for the night will depend on how awake he has been at the event, and whether he gets a second wind when you arrive home. If he has fallen asleep in the car and is very sleepy I would advise that you quickly change his nappy and put him into his night clothes before settling him, so that he goes down sleepy yet aware that he is going into his cot. If he has got a second wind and seems quite awake, implementing his normal bed- and bath-time routine should help settle him.

The important thing to remember is not to worry – whatever happens on this occasion, once back in his home environment your little one should pick up his routine again without too much trouble. I am not suggesting that you take your baby out to parties every night, but I believe that it is vital that new parents are able to enjoy themselves and maintain links with friends, and do not build up resentment for a baby who they feel is tying them to the house.

Adjusting the routines for holidays

One of the most commonly asked questions I get from parents is how to keep their baby in the routine when on holiday. Trying to have a fun and relaxing time while worrying about getting back in time for the lunchtime nap or bedtime at 7pm can be very unrelaxing. Unless you are fortunate enough to have full-time help when you are going on holiday, I would recommend you adjust the baby's routine so that you are able to go out and enjoy meals at lunchtime and in the evenings. Many of the clients I work with travel extensively, often involving long-haul flights and time differences of several hours. When travelling, I always recommend that they move their baby from the 7am-to-7pm routine to a 9–10am-to-9–10pm routine, so that the short morning nap usually comes between 11am and 12 noon, meaning that the baby is refreshed enough to go to a restaurant around 1pm to 2pm for lunch. Very young babies who are still only on milk are usually happy to sit in their buggy and observe all the hustle bustle of the restaurant; older babies will enjoy eating with their parents. I think this is much easier than trying to fit in lunch around the babies sleep time, which could result in an overtired baby not sleeping well during the lunch. The lunchtime nap then comes much later and can be done in the buggy when out and about. A lot of babies will not sleep a full two hours in the buggy after lunch, but this should not cause a problem as they will have another nap in the late afternoon anyway, so depending on which schedule your baby is on they are refreshed for dinner around 6–7pm. You may find that if your baby is under six months he may doze off in his buggy during the dinner or on the way home from the restaurant, and then wake up the minute you get back to the hotel or apartment. When this happens I used to just let the baby have a little play, then do the normal bath- and bedtime routine. I didn't get stressed that he was going to bed very late because I knew he would be sleeping much later in the morning. Sometimes a baby would be so sleepy by the time I got back to the hotel that I couldn't wake him and, if this was the case, I would usually just quickly change him into his nightclothes and give them their milk feed and settle to sleep. However, I found that they slept much better if I did manage to fit in even a quick bath and a shortened bedtime routine, as I believe that it gave the baby the signal that it was now bedtime and prepared them for the long night-time sleep. Sometimes a baby would wake up around 7–8am and when this happened I just offer a quick milk feed and settle him back to sleep until 9–10am.

Helping your baby adjust to a different time change

Because babies under a year have between one to three naps a day, I do not believe that babies suffer from the same jet lag that we adults do. When travelling on a long distance flight, I advise the parents to try and book a night flight if possible so that the baby will hopefully sleep for most of the flight. Sometimes that is not possible and if they have to do a daytime flight the important thing is to not worry too much about keeping the baby in his usual routine while travelling, and certainly don't try to keep him awake if he wants to sleep. I tend to let a baby sleep as and when he wants when travelling, although I wake him up at least an hour before landing on a long distance flight to ensure that he has had a good meal and milk feed. Regardless of where you are travelling in the world and what the time difference is, the key to avoiding having your baby awake for hours in the night is not to put them to bed until nearer 9–10pm in the evening local time. Depending on what time you arrive locally at your destination I would recommend that you adjust your baby's sleep during the day, so that they are ready to go down for a sleep of one to two hours somewhere between 6pm and 7pm. You would then wake them up and do the 5pm to 7pm routine of tea, playtime, bath time and then milk and story time somewhere between 9pm and 10pm. Sometimes a baby may wake up the first night or two, and the best way I found to deal with that was to offer a milk feed and get them back to sleep as quickly as possible. The following day, regardless of what they have done in the night, I would wake the baby somewhere between 9am and 10am, so that I could then start them on the adjusted holiday routine.

When travelling back home, I would take the same approach as on the first night, extend their day with an early evening nap so they are going to bed later, and then over a period of three days gradually wake them up a little earlier each day and put them to bed a little earlier each night until they were back on their 7am to 7pm routine.

Top Tip

The main thing is to get onto local time the minute you arrive and, apart from putting your baby to bed later the first night, don't think about the time difference. See overleaf a sample travel plan showing how to adjust the routine.

Travelling on a long-haul flight

4.40pm Give your baby a small milk feed and a good snack before you leave the house. There's not enough time to give him a proper tea before you leave and because of the time difference you want him to have a good tea later.

5.30pm Leave for the airport. Hopefully he will have a short sleep on the way to the airport, or at the airport. You need to encourage this so that he is not too tired to eat at 7.30pm.

6.30pm Arrive at airport.

7–7.30pm Give him a proper tea around this time, with a small drink of water or small drink of milk. Save his full milk feed for after take-off.

8.30pm Board plane.

9.05pm Flight departs (12 hour flight). If he has fallen asleep while waiting to board, I wouldn't wake him up for his milk feed, as I am sure at some point he will wake up on the flight and you can give him a full milk feed then. If he wakes at any time during the flight and is unsettled just offer him a milk feed and a small snack if appropriate.

Wake him up at least an hour or so before landing so that he has a good milk feed and breakfast before getting off the plane.

8.55am
(local time) Flight lands

9.45am Car transfer to hotel (45 minutes). Hopefully he will have a nap on the journey to the hotel and if not then encourage him to have a nap not long after arrival, of about 30–40 minutes. If he was awake a lot on the flight, then let him sleep for a couple of hours, but I doubt that will have happened. Try to think local time, not London time.

10.30am Arrive at hotel. If he has had a short nap earlier in the car, you should now manage to get him to fairly near what his normal routine is, so that he eating some-where around noon and ready for a longer nap. If he had a much longer morning nap, he may only have a short nap around 1pm. Regardless of what he has done earlier I would try and have him awake and feeding by around 2.30pm, so he is back on track with his routine local time.

5.00pm If he is on solids, I would offer solids around now, along with a small drink of water or a small milk feed.

6/6.30pm This is the important bit: you want him to have a nap of around 1–1½ hours. No matter how tired he may seem at this time I would not put him to bed for the night at this time, as it would mean a risk of him waking up in the middle of the night. Instead I would suggest taking him out for a walk in the buggy to get him to have a short nap.

7/7.30pm Once he has had a nap of one to one and half hours, you can wake him, offer him a small snack and keep him awake for around two hours. After he has been awake for an hour or so you can start his bed and bath routine. Watch for cues of tiredness as to when to start the bath. After the bath he needs a full milk feed, then bed at 9.30pm.

If he wakes in the night feed him quickly to get him back to sleep, count the milk he has had as his breakfast milk and go straight into solids (if he is taking them) followed by a small milk top-up for breakfast.

The following day, wake him no later than 8am local time, and adjust the routine so he has a much shorter nap in the morning, thereby getting him onto his normal routine, but sticking to local time. You will probably find that he will be ready for bed by around 7.30pm. If you want to move his routine on to 9am–9pm, let him sleep to nearer 9am.

Guide to sleep required during the first year

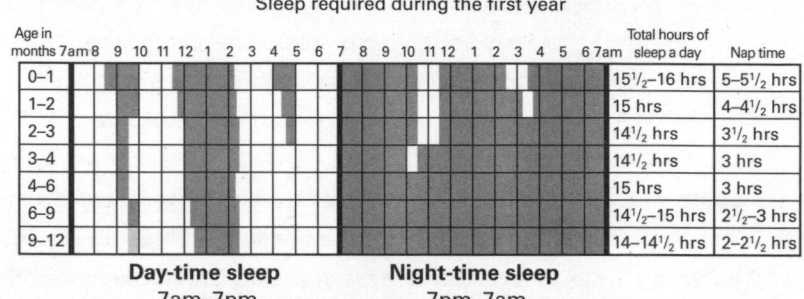

Sleep required during the first year

Age in months	7am 8 9 10 11 12 1 2 3 4 5 6 7 8 9 10 11 12 1 2 3 4 5 6 7am	Total hours of sleep a day	Nap time
0–1		$15^1/_2$–16 hrs	5–$5^1/_2$ hrs
1–2		15 hrs	4–$4^1/_2$ hrs
2–3		$14^1/_2$ hrs	$3^1/_2$ hrs
3–4		$14^1/_2$ hrs	3 hrs
4–6		15 hrs	3 hrs
6–9		$14^1/_2$–15 hrs	$2^1/_2$–3 hrs
9–12		14–$14^1/_2$ hrs	2–$2^1/_2$ hrs

Day-time sleep
7am–7pm

Night-time sleep
7pm–7am

Important recommendations

The most recent advice from The Lullaby Trust and the Department of Health on reducing risk of cot death is that, until they are six months old, babies should be put down to sleep in a room with you at all sleep times during the day and evening as well as during the night. They recommend that the safest place for a baby to sleep is in a crib, cot or Moses basket, and that babies should be checked on regularly when asleep. It is safest to have only bed clothes in the bed, and no objects like toys or muslins. They also advise that a car seat is not an ideal place for very young babies to sleep in the home, and that on long car journeys babies should be carefully observed while in the car seat, with regular stops for fresh air and feeding.

It is also important to remember that these recommendations are only for the first six months, and that after that time you can start to settle your baby in his own room for naps and night-time sleep. Until your baby reaches six months, you will have to alter the bedtime routine after his bath, so that you can finish off the remainder of the bedtime routine in the room where the baby is being settled to sleep for the evening. Try to replicate the same atmosphere here as you would in his bedroom by keeping everything calm and quiet. It is unlikely that you will have a cot in your living room, therefore, according to The Lullaby Trust, a pram with a proper mattress would be an acceptable option. (Throughout this book, in all routines up to six months, I refer to your baby's place of sleep as his 'bed', which could be a pram or cot.)

It is important to follow the same guidelines for settling your baby in the pram as those given for you settling your baby in a cot. The baby should be placed in the pram with his feet at the bottom and it is essential that any sheets and blankets used are tucked in securely so that they cannot work their way loose. Please see page 7, check the images on The Lullaby Trust's website or the sleep video at contentedbaby.com on how to do this properly. The Lullaby Trust understands that, during the day and evening, there will be times when a baby is asleep and parents may have to leave the room for a short spell. They say this is acceptable as long as the baby is not left for lengthy periods on his own while asleep. If you have any concerns about this advice it is important that you contact The Lullaby Trust or discuss them with your health visitor or GP.

Although the new guidelines may mean that it will take a little longer to establish the routines, please take heart that your baby will eventually get into a good sleep routine and sleep right through the night.

6

Weeks One to Two

Starting the routine

The following checklist will help you decide if your baby is ready to move on from feeding three-hourly into the one- to two-week routine:

- Your baby has regained his birth weight.

- He is happily going three hours between feeds, the three hours being calculated from the beginning of one feed to the beginning of the next feed. This means that if a feed has been taking around one hour, there is only a two-hour gap between feeds.

- Your baby shows signs of wanting to go longer between some feeds – you have to wake him for some of his feeds.

- He is staying awake happily for a short time after some of his feeds.

If your baby is showing all of the above signs, you can confidently start to implement the one- to two-week routine. The one- to two-week routine is not so different to the three-hourly routine, except that it starts to establish proper nap times, in particular the lunchtime nap. It is also the beginning of you starting to introduce a proper bedtime routine, and a longer sleep after the bedtime bath. Your baby will still need to be fed three-hourly at some parts of the day, but in the one- to two-week routine there is a split feed at 10–11.15am in the morning, which helps establish the lunchtime nap. This routine also includes a split feed at 5–6.15pm, which will help encourage a longer sleep between 7pm and 10pm.

When moving on through the routines, it is important to remember that your baby's feeding and sleeping needs may not automatically fit straight into the feeding and sleeping times of the next routine. Some babies go through a stage of needing one routine for feeding but a different one for sleeping.

Starting the routine with premature babies

If your baby had been born prematurely you will probably find that by the time he leaves the hospital he will already be in a regular feeding routine, as it is essential with premature babies that they are not allowed to go long spells between feeds. Usually I found that the babies were feeding three hourly around the clock, and parents were advised to do this until the babies reached somewhere between 2.7–3.2kg (6–7lbs) in weight. At this point they were normally advised that the baby could then be left to sleep a longer spell after the late feed. It is important that you check with your GP or health visitor at what age you can stop waking your baby for a feed in the night. I would recommend that you continue on the Week One routine until your baby shows signs of starting to be more awake and alert after feeds. Once he is managing to stay awake happily for nearer an hour, you could then move onto the Two to Four Week routine. Another sign that your baby may be ready to stay awake a bit longer during the day after feeds is if he starts to become very awake during the night feeds. The most important thing I found with premature babies is not to reduce the number of feeds too quickly. By feeding them enough so that each week they put on more than the recommended weight expected of a full term baby, meant that by three to four months their weight was near enough as close to what a full-term baby's weight was, and they were then able to follow the routine for that age.

Starting the routine with older babies

If you are starting the routine with an older baby, look through the routines nearest to his age and start on the one that is closest to what he is doing at the moment. You may find that you have to start with a routine for a baby a few weeks younger; this is not a problem as once you have him established on that routine, and his night-time sleep improves, you can very quickly move him onto a routine suitable for his age. If your baby has been used to being fed on demand and rocked to sleep or has developed the wrong sleep associations, you may find that he fights sleep at the times recommended in the routine as he is not used to self-settling. If this happens I would recommend that you use the Assisting to sleep method on page 337. It is a gentle way of getting him into the habit of self-settling at sleep times.

Routine – one to two weeks

Feed times	Nap times between 7am and 7pm
7am	8.15–8.30–10am
10am	11.30am–2–2.30pm
11–11.15am	3.30–5pm
2–2.30pm	
5pm	
6–6.15pm	
10–11.15pm	Maximum daily sleep: 5–6 hours

Expressing times: 7.30am and 10.45am

7am

- Baby should be awake, nappy changed and feeding no later than 7am.

- He needs up to 20–30 minutes from the full breast, then offer 10–15 minutes from the breast that you have expressed 90ml (3oz) from.

- If he fed at 5am or 6am, offer up to 15–20 minutes from the second breast after expressing 90ml (3oz).

- Do not feed baby after 8am, as it will put him off his next feed.

- He can stay awake for up to one and a half hours.

- Make sure you get some breakfast no later than 8am while baby has a kick on his play mat.

8.15am

- Baby should start to get a bit sleepy by this time. Even if he does not show the signs, he will be getting tired, so check his nappy and start winding down now.
- Wash and dress baby, remembering to cream all of his creases.

8.15–8.30am

- When he is drowsy, settle baby in his bed, fully swaddled (see page 27), no later than 8.30am.

- Wash and sterilise any bottles and expressing equipment.

9.45am

- Unswaddle baby so that he can wake up naturally.

- Prepare things for dressing.

10am

- Baby must be fully awake now, regardless of how long he slept.

- He should be given up to 20–30 minutes from the breast he last fed on, while you drink a large glass of water.

- Lay him on his play mat so that he can have a good kick, while you prepare equipment for expressing.

10.45am

- Express 60ml (2oz) from the second breast.

11–11.15am

- Baby should start to get a bit sleepy by this time. Even if he does not show the signs, he will be getting tired, so change his nappy and start winding down now.

- Offer baby up to 15–20 minutes from the breast you last expressed from.

- When he is drowsy, settle baby in his bed, fully swaddled, no later than 11.30am.

- If he doesn't settle within 10 minutes, offer him up to 10 minutes from the fuller breast. Do this with no talking or eye contact.

11.30am–2pm

- Baby needs a total nap time of no longer than two and a half to three hours from the time he went down.

- If he wakes up after 45 minutes, check the swaddle, but do not overstimulate him with lots of talking or eye contact.

- Allow 10 minutes for him to resettle himself; if he's still unsettled, offer him half his 2–2.30pm feed and try to settle him back to sleep until 2.30pm.

12 noon

- Wash and sterilise expressing equipment, then you should have lunch and a rest before the next feed.

2–2.30pm

- Baby must be awake and feeding no later than 2.30pm, regardless of how long he has slept.

- Unswaddle him and allow him to wake naturally. Change his nappy.

- Give him up to 20–30 minutes from the breast he last fed on. If he is still hungry, offer up to 10–15 minutes from the other breast while you drink a large glass of water.

- Try not to feed baby after 3.15pm, as this could put him off his next feed.

- It is very important that he is fully awake now as near to 3.30pm as possible, so he goes down well at 7pm; if he was very alert in the morning, he may be sleepier now. Do not overdress him, as extra warmth will make him drowsy.

3.30pm

- Change baby's nappy.

- Baby needs a nap of up to one and a half hours. This is a good time to take him for a walk to ensure that he naps well and is refreshed for his next feed and bath.

- Baby should not sleep after 5pm if you want him to go down well at 7pm.

5pm

- Baby must be fully awake and feeding no later than 5pm.

- Give him up to 20–30 minutes from the breast he last fed on, while you drink a large glass of water.

- It is very important that he is not dozy while feeding (see page 324) and that he waits for the other breast until after his bath.

5.45pm

- If baby has been very wakeful during the day or didn't nap well between 3.30pm and 5pm, he may need to start his bath and next feed earlier so he can be in bed by 6.30pm.

- Allow baby a good kick without his nappy while you prepare things needed for his bath and bedtime.

- Baby must start his bath no later than 5.45pm, and be massaged and dressed by 6–6.15pm.

6–6.15pm

- Baby must be feeding no later than 6.15pm; this should be done in a quiet, dimly lit room with care taken not to over-stimulate him with lots of talking or eye contact.

- If he did not finish the first breast at 5pm, give him up to 5–10 minutes from it before putting him on the second breast. Allow up to 15–20 minutes from the second breast.

- It is very important that baby is in bed two hours from when he last woke. Some babies may need to be in bed by 6.30pm.

6.30–7pm

- When drowsy, settle baby in his bed, fully swaddled, no later than 7pm.

- If baby hasn't settled well, offer him up to 10 minutes from the fuller breast. Do this without overstimulating him with lots of talking or eye contact.

8pm

- It is very important that you have a really good meal and a rest before the next feed.

9.45pm

- Turn up the lights fully and unswaddle baby so that he can wake up naturally. Allow at least 10 minutes before feeding to ensure that he is fully awake and can feed well.

- Lay out things for the nappy change, plus a spare draw sheet, muslin and swaddle blanket in case they are needed in the middle of the night.

10pm

- Give baby up to 20–30 minutes from the breast he last fed on, or most of his bottle-feed, change his nappy and re-swaddle him.

- Dim the lights and, with no talking or eye contact, give him up to 15–30 minutes on the second breast or the remainder of his bottle-feed.

- It is important that your baby is awake for a full hour at this stage.

In the night

- During this week, it is important that breast-fed babies are not allowed to go too long in the night between feeds.

- A baby weighing less than 3.2kg (7lb) at birth should be woken at around 2.30am for a feed, and a baby weighing between 3.2–3.6kg (7–8lb) should be woken no later than 3.30am.

- A formula-fed baby who weighs more than 3.6kg (8lb) or a baby that weighed over 3.6kg (8lb) at birth, who has fed well during the day, may be able to go slightly longer, but not longer than five hours.

- If you are in doubt as to how long to allow your baby to sleep between feeds in the night, please seek advice from your GP or health visitor.

Changes to be made during the one- to two-week routine

Sleeping

Depending on how long your baby sleeps after the late feed, you can choose one of the following options:

- If your baby feeds and settles well and then sleeps until after 2am, then feeds well in the night and sleeps until nearer 6am, following the routine and having him awake for an hour at the late feed is fine.

- If your baby feeds well and settles well after being awake for an hour at the late feed, but then wakes up before 2am and then wakes up again before 6am, I would recommend splitting the late feed to try to eliminate the twice-a-night waking. It can take at least a week to establish this split feed so do not get disheartened if you do not see immediate results. For the split feed to work well, you should start to wake your baby at around 9.45pm, and by 10pm start the feed. Give him as much of this feed as he wants, then allow him to have a good kick on his play mat. At nearer 11pm take him to the bedroom, change his nappy, then offer him the second part of his feed. If he is formula-fed, I would advise that you make up two bottles.

Most babies in the early days can stay awake happily for up to two hours before needing a nap. This does not mean they *must* stay awake for the full two hours, only that it is important that they do not stay awake for longer than two hours if overtiredness is to be avoided. So if, during the early days, you find that your baby is only staying awake for an hour or an hour and a half at a time, providing he is sleeping well at night, you do not need to worry as he is obviously a baby that needs more sleep, and as he grows he will start to stay awake longer (see page 110).

Feeding

When your baby wakes in the night, it is really important that he takes a big enough feed, so that he sleeps well until nearer 6–7am. You should not restrict the amount he wants to feed at this stage; by doing so you could risk him waking at 5am looking for another feed. At this stage you are aiming to feed your baby well enough so that he only needs to feed once between 11pm and 6–7am.

- Depending on what time he fed in the night, your baby will probably wake up between 6am and 7am, but he should always be woken at 7am regardless. If he wakes up at 6am, this means that you can give him most of his first morning feed (treat this as a night feed), and then offer him a top-up feed between 7–8am. He may then need another top-up feed just prior to his morning map.

- During this routine I suggest that you always offer the baby a top-up feed at 11–11.15am, or just prior to the lunchtime nap. This will hopefully avoid him waking up hungry during the middle of the nap. However, should he wake up before 2pm, I would assume that hunger is the genuine cause and offer him a feed before trying to settle him back to sleep until 2.30pm. If he will not settle back to sleep, then it is best just to get him up, and then offer him two shorter naps at around 2.30pm and 4–4.30pm.

Moving on to the two- to four-week routine

By the end of the second week, you may be able to advance on to the two- to four-week routine.

The following signs will help you decide whether your baby is ready to advance on to the two- to four-week routine:

- Your baby should weigh over 3.2kg (7lb), have regained his birth weight and be gaining weight steadily.

- He is sleeping well at nap times and more often than not you have to wake him from his naps for him to be fed.

- He is feeding more efficiently and often finishing a breast-feed within 25–30 minutes.

- He is showing signs of being more alert and managing to stay awake easily for an hour and a half at a time.

If you find that your baby is happy to go longer between feeds, but still needs to sleep more than the two- to four-week routine suggests, then you can still follow this routine for feeding, and continue to follow the one- to two-week routine for sleep until he shows signs of needing less sleep. Remember that a baby who needs more sleep will be sleeping well at night as well as during the day. If your baby is sleeping well during the day, but starting to be more wakeful in the middle of the night, it is possibly a sign he needs to be awake more during the day. By settling him for some of his naps one or two minutes later each day, you will gradually extend the time he is awake without him getting overtired.

7

Weeks Two to Four

Routine – two to four weeks

Feed times	Nap times between 7am and 7pm
7am	8.30–10am
10am	11.30am/12 noon–2–2.30pm
11.30–11.45am	4–5pm
2–2.30pm	
5pm	
6–6.15pm	
10–10.30pm	Maximum daily sleep: 5 hours

Expressing times: 7.30am, 10.30am and 9.30pm

7am

- Baby should be awake, nappy changed and feeding no later than 7am.

- If he fed before 5am, he needs up to 15–25 minutes from the full breast, then offer up to 10–15 minutes from the breast that you have expressed approximately 60–90ml (2–3oz) from.

- If he fed at 5am or 6am, offer up to 20–25 minutes from the second breast after expressing 90ml (3oz).

- Do not feed baby after 8am, as it will put him off his next feed.

- He can stay awake for up to two hours.

- Try to have some cereal, toast and a drink no later than 8am while baby has a kick on his play mat.

- Wash and dress him, remembering to cream all his creases and dry skin.

8.30

- Baby should start to get a bit sleepy by this time. Even if he does not show the signs, he will be getting tired, so start winding down now.

- When he is drowsy, settle baby in his bed, fully swaddled, no later than 9am. He needs a nap of no longer than one and a half hours.

- Wash and sterilise bottles and expressing equipment.

9.45am

- Unswaddle baby so that he can wake up naturally.

- Prepare things for top-and-tailing and dressing.

10am

- Baby must be fully awake now, regardless of how long he slept.

- He should be given up to 20–25 minutes from the breast he last fed on, while you drink a large glass of water.

10.30am

- Lay baby on his play mat so that he can have a good kick while you express 60ml (2oz) from the second breast.

11.30am

- If baby was very alert and awake during the previous two hours, he may start to get tired by 11.15am and would need to be in bed by 11.30am.

- Offer baby up to 15 minutes from the breast you last expressed from, immediately prior to going for his nap.

11.45am

- Regardless of what baby has done earlier, he should now be winding down for his nap.

- Check the draw sheet and change his nappy.

- When he is drowsy, settle baby in his bed, fully swaddled, no later than 12 noon.

11.30am/12 noon–2pm

- Baby needs a total nap time of no longer than two and a half hours from the time he went down.

- If he slept one and a half hours earlier, only allow him two hours this nap time.

- If he wakes up after 30–45 minutes, check the swaddle, but do not overstimulate him with lots of talking or eye contact.

- Allow 10 minutes or so for him to resettle himself; if he's still unsettled, offer him half his 2–2.30pm feed and try to settle him back to sleep until 2.30pm. If he doesn't settle back to sleep, get him up and do a split afternoon nap (see page 137) so you can keep him on track for a 7pm bedtime.

12–12.30pm

- Wash and sterilise expressing equipment, then you should have lunch and a rest before the next feed.

2pm–2.30pm

- Baby must be awake and feeding no later than 2–2.30pm, regardless of how long he has slept.

- Unswaddle him and allow him to wake naturally. Change his nappy.

- Give him up to 20–25 minutes from the breast he last fed on. If he is still hungry, offer up to 10–15 minutes from the other breast, while you drink a large glass of water.

- Try not to feed baby after 3.15pm as it will put him off his next feed.

- If he had a broken lunchtime nap and didn't settle back to sleep, he will need to have a short cat-nap of 20 minutes fairly soon after his feed. He will then be ready for another nap around 4.30pm. By splitting the nap you will ensure that he doesn't sleep too much in the afternoon, which could result in him not settling well at 7pm.

- If he slept well at the lunchtime nap, it is very important that he is fully awake now until as near 4pm, so he goes down well at 7pm; if he was very alert in the morning, he may be sleepier now. Do not overdress him, as extra warmth will make him drowsy.

- Lay baby on his play mat and encourage him to have a good kick.

3.45–4pm

- Change baby's nappy.

- This is a good time to take him for a walk to ensure that he naps well, and is refreshed for his next feed and bath.

- Baby should not sleep after 5pm if you want him to go down well at 7pm.

5pm

- Baby must be fully awake and feeding no later than 5pm.

- Give him up to 20 minutes from the breast he last fed on, while you drink a large glass of water.

- It is very important that he waits for the other breast until after his bath.

5.45pm

- If baby has been very wakeful during the day, or didn't nap well between 4pm and 5pm, he may need to start his bath and next feed early.

- Allow baby a good kick without his nappy, while you prepare things needed for his bath and bedtime.

- Baby must start his bath no later than 6pm, and be massaged and dressed by 6.15pm.

6–6.15pm

- Baby must be feeding no later than 6.15pm; this should be done in a quiet, dimly lit room with care taken not to over-stimulate him with lots of talking or eye contact.

- If he did not finish the first breast at 5pm, give him up to 5–10 minutes from it before putting him on the second breast. Allow up to 20–25 minutes from the second breast.

- It is very important that baby is in bed two hours from when he last woke.

6.30–7pm

- When he is drowsy, settle baby in his bed, fully swaddled, no later than 7pm.

- If baby hasn't settled well, offer him up to 10–15 minutes from the fuller breast. Do this without overstimulating him with lots of talking or eye contact.

8pm

- It is very important that you have a really good meal and a rest before the next feed or expressing.

9.30pm

- If you have chosen to replace the late feed with a bottle feed, then express from both breasts now.

10–10.30pm

- Turn up the lights fully and unswaddle baby so that he can wake up naturally. Allow at least 10 minutes before feeding to ensure he is fully awake, so that he can feed well.

- Lay out things for the nappy change, plus a spare draw sheet, muslin and swaddle blanket in case they are needed in the middle of the night.

- Give baby up to 20 minutes from the breast he last fed on, or most of his bottle-feed, change his nappy and re-swaddle him.

- Dim the lights and, with no talking or eye contact, give him up to 20 minutes from the second breast or the remainder of the bottle-feed.

- It is important that your baby is awake for a full hour at this stage.

In the night

- If baby wakes between 2am and 4am, it is important that you give him a big enough feed to help him sleep nearer 7am. If he falls asleep after feeding from one breast, and then he is waking again at 5am, it is worth trying to get him slightly more awake so that he feeds from both breasts.

- If he wakes between 4am and 5am, give him one breast, then start the 7am feed on the fuller breast.

- If he wakes at 6am, give him one breast, then the second at 7.30am after expressing.

- Keep the lights low and do not overstimulate him with lots of talking or eye contact. Only change his nappy if absolutely necessary, or if he is too sleepy to take a full feed.

Changes to be made during the two- to four-week routine

The two- to four-week routine usually coincides with your baby's first growth spurt. Many babies become a bit fretful or unsettled during growth spurts, so even if your partner has gone back to work full-time, try to arrange for him to get home earlier than usual, if possible, so that he can help out with the bedtime routine. The majority of babies get a bit irritable around 5pm and it is probably the most challenging time of the day for all mothers, so do not take it as a failure on your part if things get fraught at this time of the day.

Sleeping

By three to four weeks, your baby should start to show signs of being more wakeful and for longer periods. Ensure that you encourage the wakefulness during the day so that his night-time sleep is not affected. It is really important to ensure that your baby is fully awake while feeding. One of the main reasons why babies of this age start to fight sleep or do not sleep well at nap times is because they have been sleepy feeding on the breast.

- By four weeks aim for the morning nap to be no more than one hour, to ensure that he sleeps well at lunchtime. Gradually, aim to keep him awake longer in the morning, until he is going down for his sleep at 9am. If you find that he is going to sleep at 8.30am and waking up between 9.15am and 9.30am, which has an adverse effect on the rest of the day, refer to page 137 on how to implement a split nap to get the routine on track for the lunch time nap.

- The afternoon nap should be no more than one hour in total; this nap is sometimes broken into a couple of catnaps between 4pm and 5pm. By four weeks he should be half-swaddled, under the arms (see page 27), for the morning and for the late afternoon nap. Around four weeks it becomes more obvious when the baby comes into his light sleep: normally every 45 minutes, although it can be every 30 minutes with some babies. If a feed is not due, most babies, given the opportunity, settle themselves back to sleep. Rushing too quickly to your baby and assisting him back to sleep by rocking could result in a long-term sleep association problem. This means that in the night when your baby comes into his light sleep, you could end up getting up several times to help him back to sleep, long after the time he no longer needs night feeds.

- If you find that settling your baby at naps is becoming a real issue I would recommend that, for a few days, you top him up before each nap with a small milk feed to eliminate the possibility of hunger being the cause. If he then settles and sleeps well, hunger is probably the cause. If you are breast-feeding, offering a top-up for several days should help to increase your milk supply. You can then start to decrease gradually the time you offer him on the breast until the top-up is eliminated altogether. At this point you would need to encourage him to drink more at his original feed, if you do not want him to return to being unsettled at nap times.

- With bottle-fed babies you can try offering one or two ounces (30–60mls) of milk just prior to naps, and once he settles well again, the top-up should be brought back gradually nearer to his feed time until the original feed and top-up is being done within one hour and the amount he drinks is being increased.

Feeding

Most babies go through a growth spurt around the third week. When your baby goes through a growth spurt, reduce the amount you express at 7.30am by 30ml (1oz) and by the end of the fourth week reduce the 10.30am expressing by 30ml (1oz). This will ensure that your baby immediately receives the extra milk he needs.

- If you have not been expressing, you will need to allow your baby to feed more often on the breast and for longer periods, in order for him to get the amounts he needs. During this time, try to get extra rest so that your baby's increased feeding demands do not have the opposite effect on you, causing you to become so exhausted that your milk supply decreases even further.

- If you think low milk supply is a problem in the evening, try using the plan on page 313, which increases your milk supply without losing the sleep routine. Once your milk supply has increased, you can then go back to following the routine suitable for your baby's age. Continuing to split the mid-morning feed and offering the baby a top-up of milk immediately prior to the lunchtime nap should help him sleep well here.

- If you are breast-feeding and have decided to give one bottle-feed a day, this is a good age to introduce it. If you leave it any later than this age, it is very possible that your baby will refuse a bottle altogether, which can cause enormous problems later on, particularly if you are going back to work.

- If you are replacing the late feed with a bottle feed, it is advisable to express between 9.30pm and 10pm, extracting as much milk as possible, as this will help keep your milk supply up. This milk can either be used for the late feed, or frozen and used on the occasions when you need to leave your baby with a babysitter. Introducing a bottle of expressed milk at the late feed also allows your partner to get involved and enables you to get to bed earlier, giving you the extra sleep that all mothers need during the early weeks.

- If you wish to breast-feed for longer than six weeks, avoid giving formula at any other feeds, unless advised to do so by your health visitor or GP.

- Bottle-fed babies should have their 7am, 10am and late feeds increased first during growth spurts. Some bottle-fed babies are ready to go from using a newborn teat to the next size up (see next page).

- Low weight gain in breast-fed babies is usually caused by a low milk supply or poor positioning at the breast; the two often go hand in hand. It would be worthwhile following the plan for increasing your milk supply on page 313. I would also advise that you arrange a home visit from a breast-feeding counsellor to check that you are positioning your baby on the breast correctly. If your baby is formula-fed and not gaining sufficient weight, try moving him from the newborn teat with one hole to the slow flow teat with two holes. Always discuss any concerns you have regarding your baby's low weight gain with your health visitor or GP.

- If you find your baby is still waking at around 2am then again at 5am, I would suggest that you introduce a split feed at the late feed. Start to wake him up at 9.45pm, so that he is wide awake by 10pm. Give him most of his feed and keep him awake for longer than the recommended one hour. At 11.15pm his nappy should be changed and the lights dimmed while you give him a small top-up feed. By giving him a split feed and having him awake slightly longer at this time, he will more than likely sleep well past 3am, provided he is not getting out of his swaddle.

- Once your baby reaches four weeks, he will probably show signs of being happy to go slightly longer between feeds, and you should be able to move him on to the four- to six-week feeding routine, provided he is gaining weight steadily. Babies who are not gaining sufficient weight should remain on the two- to four-week routine until their weight gain improves.

- In my experience, babies who regularly gain between 170–226g (6–8oz) a week in the first few months are usually more content and sleep better than those who are putting on less than 140g (5oz) a week. On saying this, I have cared for some very happy and contented babies who would thrive well on a weight gain of only 110–140g (4–5oz) a week. However, if you find your baby is constantly irritable between feeds, not sleeping well at night and gaining less than 170g (6oz) a week, it may be that he is not getting enough to eat and it would be advisable to discuss his weight gain with your health visitor or GP.

8

Weeks Four to Six

Routine – four to six weeks

Feed times	Nap times between 7am and 7pm
7am	9–10am
10.30am	11.30am/12 noon–2–2.30pm
2–2.30pm	4.15pm–5pm
5pm	6–6.15pm
10–10.30pm	Maximum daily sleep: $4\frac{3}{4}$ hours

Expressing times: 7.30am, 10.30am and 9.30pm

7am

- Baby should be awake, nappy changed and feeding no later than 7am.

- If he fed before 5am, he needs up to 20–25 minutes from the full breast. If he's still hungry, offer up to 10–15 minutes from the breast that you have expressed approximately 60ml (2oz) from.

- If he fed at 5am or 6am, offer up to 20–25 minutes from the second breast after expressing approximately 60ml (2oz).

- Do not feed baby after 8am, as it will put him off his next feed.

- He can stay awake for up to two hours.

- Try to have some breakfast no later than 8am while baby has a kick on his play mat.

- Wash and dress him, remembering to cream all his creases and dry skin.

8.45–9 am

- Baby should start to get a bit sleepy by this time. Even if he does not show the signs, he will be getting tired, so check his nappy and draw sheet and start winding down now.

- When he is drowsy, settle baby in his bed, fully or half-swaddled (see page 27), no later than 9am. He needs a nap of no longer than one hour.

- Wash and sterilise bottles and expressing equipment.

9.45am

- Unswaddle baby so that he can wake up naturally.

- Prepare things for top-and-tailing and dressing.

10am

- Baby must be fully awake now, regardless of how long he slept.

10.30am

- Baby should be given up to 20–25 minutes from the breast he last fed on, while you drink a large glass of water.

- Lay him on his play mat so that he can have a good kick while you express 30ml (1oz) from the second breast. Then offer him up to 10–15 minutes from this breast.

11.30am

- If baby was very alert and awake during the previous two hours, he may start to get tired by 11.30am and would need to be in bed by 11.45am.

11.45am

- Regardless of what baby has done earlier, he should now be winding down for his nap.

- Check the draw sheet and change his nappy.

- When he is drowsy, settle baby in his bed, fully swaddled, no later than 12 noon.

12 noon–2–2.30pm

- Baby needs a nap of no longer than two and a half hours from the time he went down.

- If he wakes up after 45 minutes, check the swaddle, but do not overstimulate him with lots of talking or eye contact.

- Allow 10–20 minutes for him to resettle himself; if he's still unsettled, offer him half his 2pm feed and try to settle him back to sleep until 2pm.

- If he does not go back to sleep you will need to give him a short catnap after his next feed so that he gets through happily until his afternoon nap.

12 noon

- Wash and sterilise expressing equipment, then you should have lunch and a rest before the next feed.

2–2.30pm

- Baby must be awake and feeding no later than 2.30pm, regardless of how long he has slept.

- Unswaddle him and allow him to wake naturally. Change his nappy.

- Give him up to 20–25 minutes from the breast he last fed on. If he is still hungry, offer him up to 10–15 minutes from the other breast, while you drink a large glass of water.

- Do not feed baby after 3.15pm as it will put him off his next feed.

- It is very important that he is fully awake now until nearer 4.15pm, so he goes down well at 7pm; if he was very alert in the morning, he may be sleepier now. Do not overdress him, as extra warmth will make him drowsy.

- Lay baby on his play mat and encourage him to have a good kick.

4–4.15pm

- Change baby's nappy.

- This is a good time to take him for a walk to ensure that he naps well, and is refreshed for his next feed and bath. He may start to cut right back on this nap or catnap on and off.

- Baby should not sleep after 5pm if you want him to go down well at 7pm.

5pm

- Baby must be fully awake and feeding no later than 5pm.

- Give him up to 20 minutes from the breast he last fed on, while you drink a large glass of water.

- It is very important that he waits for the other breast until after his bath.

5.45pm

- If baby has been very wakeful during the day, or didn't nap well between 4.15pm and 5pm, he may need to start his bath and next feed early.

- Allow baby a good kick without his nappy while you prepare things needed for his bath and bedtime.

6pm

- Baby must start his bath no later than 6pm, and be massaged and dressed by 6.15pm.

6.15pm

- Baby must be feeding no later than 6.15pm; this should be done in a quiet, dimly lit room with care taken not to over-stimulate him with lots of talking or eye contact.

- If he did not finish the first breast at 5pm, give him up to 5–10 minutes from it before putting him on the second breast. Allow up to 20–25 minutes from the full breast.

- It is very important that baby is in bed two hours from when he last woke.

7pm

- When he is drowsy, settle baby in his bed, fully swaddled, no later than 7pm.

- If baby hasn't settled well, offer him up to 10 minutes from the fuller breast. Do this without overstimulating him with lots of talking or eye contact.

8pm

- It is very important that you have a really good meal and a rest before the next feed or expressing.

9.30pm

- If you have chosen to replace the late feed with a bottle feed, then express from both breasts now.

10–10.30pm

- Turn up the lights fully and unswaddle baby so that he can wake up naturally. Allow at least 10 minutes before feeding to ensure that he is fully awake, so that he can feed well.

- Lay out things for the nappy change, plus a spare draw sheet, muslin and swaddle blanket in case they are needed in the middle of the night.

- Give baby up to 20 minutes from the breast he last fed from or most of his bottle-feed, change his nappy and re-swaddle him.

- Dim the lights and, with no talking or eye contact, give him up to 20 minutes from the second breast or the remainder of the bottle-feed.
- It is important that your baby is awake for a full hour at this stage.

In the night

- If baby wakes up before 4am, give him a full feed.

- If he wakes between 4am and 5am, give one breast, then start the 7am feed on the fuller breast.

- If he wakes up at 6am, give him one breast, then the second at 7.30am after expressing.

- Keep the lights low and do not overstimulate him with lots of talking or eye contact. Only change his nappy if absolutely necessary, or if he is too sleepy to take a full feed.

Changes to be made during the four- to six-week routine

Sleeping

By the age of six weeks, the majority of babies that I cared for were sleeping for a much longer spell during the night, and many were sleeping through to nearer 7am. Parents who are struggling to get their babies to sleep longer often ask me how I achieved this. My response has always been that, by following the routines, it just happened naturally, and that the babies themselves started to sleep longer and longer in the night. Certainly from reading the forums on my website, this seems to be true for the majority of parents. But what has also become obvious from reading thousands of posts over the last few years is that many of the parents whose babies do not manage to sleep a longer stretch during the night by six weeks appear to have much more sleep during the day than I recommend at this age. They believe that they have sleepy babies that need more daytime sleep. While I do believe that some babies need more sleep, from my own personal experience those babies who genuinely needed more sleep would also begin to sleep longer in the night.

- If your baby is not showing signs of sleeping longer during the night, perhaps look more closely at his daytime sleep, and gradually start to reduce the amount he is having. By putting him down for his first nap of the day a couple of minutes later every three or four days, it will avoid the problem of him becoming overtired and not settling, but also reduce the amount of daytime sleep he is having.

- I recommend that at this stage the daily nap time between 7am and 7pm should be reduced to around four and a half hours: the morning nap should be no more than one hour and the afternoon nap no more than 30 minutes between 4.15pm and 5pm. Some babies tend to doze off at around 8.30am, and then sleep until nearer 10am; this results in too much daytime sleep and can affect how long the baby sleeps at night or the lunchtime nap.

- If you find your baby is falling asleep around 8.30am, I would recommend that you introduce a split nap for a short spell. This will help him get through the morning happily to the lunchtime nap and also eliminate the chance of him having too much daytime sleep. To implement the split morning nap, I would suggest that after 20–30 minutes you wake your baby up at 9am, then allow him a further 10–15 minute catnap between 10.30 and 11am. He should be fully awake by 11am. This will keep his total morning sleep to just under an hour, and by allowing only a 10–15 minute nap his lunchtime nap should not be affected.

- It is very important that by the end of six weeks you start to get your baby used to being half-swaddled (under the arms) for the 9am and the 7pm naps. Cot death rates peak between two and four months and overheating is considered to be a major factor in this.

- When you start to half-swaddle your baby, it is important to tuck him in securely. If he is waking earlier than the time the routine suggests, check if he has kicked his covers off; babies become more active at this age and this is another cause of them waking up earlier in the night. For advice on how to securely tuck in your baby, and prevent him from doing this, see page 7.

- It should now take less time to settle your baby to sleep. The cuddling time should gradually be reduced and now is a good time to get him used to going down when he is more awake. Often a lullaby light, which plays a tune and casts images on the ceiling for 10 minutes or so, will help a baby to settle himself.

- Another important factor in helping your baby sleep longer in the night is to ensure that he is getting most of his daily milk intake between 6–7am and 11.30pm. A good indicator of this will be his weight gain; he should be gaining weight steadily. See page 186 for information on weight gain.

- Once he has slept a longer stretch several nights in a row, try not to feed him if he suddenly goes back to waking earlier again. The hours after the late feed are sometimes referred to as the 'core night' (see page 322 for a full explanation of the 'core night method'). On waking at this time, he should initially be left for a few minutes to settle himself back to sleep. If that doesn't work, then other methods apart from feeding should be used to settle him. I would try settling him with a cuddle. Attention should be kept to the minimum, while reassuring your baby that you are there. This teaches the baby one of the most important sleep skills: how to go back to sleep after surfacing from a non-REM sleep. Obviously, if he refuses to settle you would need to feed him.

- The core night method could also be used to encourage an older baby who has got into the habit of waking at the same time in the night to sleep longer. Before embarking on this method, the following points should be read carefully to make sure that your baby really is capable of going for a longer spell in the night:

    - These methods should never be used with a very small baby or a baby who is not gaining weight.

    - The above methods should only be used if your baby is gaining weight steadily, and if you are sure that his last feed is substantial enough to help him sleep for the longer stretch in the night.

    - The main sign that a baby is ready to cut down on a night feed is regular weight gain and taking only a very small feed in the middle of the night and sleeping nearer to 7am.

    - The aim of this method is gradually to increase the length of time your baby can go from his last feed and not to eliminate the night feed in one go. The core night method can be used if, over three or four nights, a baby has shown signs that he is capable of sleeping for a longer stretch. However, I cannot stress enough the importance of not using this method if your baby is not settling quickly in the night. If it is not working within three or four nights, you should abandon it and continue to feed your baby. If you persist with this method and your baby is not settling back quickly, you will actually create a sleep association problem that could mean your baby will continue to be unsettled in the night for many weeks.

Feeding

If your baby is feeding between 3am and 4am, you have to wake him up at 7am every morning for at least 10 days and he is starting to show less interest in his morning feed, then you can very gradually, and by a small amount, cut back the amount of milk he is taking in the night. This will have the knock-on effect of him drinking more during the day and less in the night, and eventually he will drop the middle-of-the-night feed altogether. It is important not to cut back too much or too fast as the baby could then start to wake up hungry long before 7am; this will defeat the whole purpose of getting him to sleep through from 11pm to 6–7am.

- At around six weeks, your baby will go through another growth spurt, and you will need to reduce the amount you are expressing first thing in the morning by a further 30ml (1oz), and cut out the mid-morning expressing altogether. If your baby woke and fed well between 3am and 4am, slept until 7am, then woke and fed well again, he should be happy to go a longer stretch after the 7am feed.

- You can gradually start to push the 10am feed to nearer 10.30am. The exception to this would be a baby who is getting to nearer 5am in the morning and having a top-up between 7–8am. It is unlikely that he would get through to 10.30am if he's only had a top-up feed at 7.30am, so continue to feed him at 10am (with a top-up prior to the lunchtime nap) until he is feeding nearer to 7am.

- During growth spurts, your baby will probably need to spend longer on the breast at some feeds, especially if you have not been expressing at the suggested times. It is important to allow the baby this extra time on the breast and, if need be, additional top-ups. While it may feel as if you are backtracking with the routines, the extra feeding during the day will only be short term, and will avoid the problem of your baby starting to wake up earlier or more in the night because he has not fed well enough during the day or at the bedtime or late feeds. For a plan to increase your milk supply see page 313.

- Bottle-fed babies should have the 7am, the 10.30am and the 6.15pm feeds increased first during growth spurts. However it is important not to increase the 6.15pm feed so much that it reduces your baby's appetite for his late feed. Some babies may also need their late feed increased.

- If your baby is happily waiting until 10.30am for his feed, and during this growth spurt you find that he starts to wake up during his lunchtime nap or earlier than usual, it would be worthwhile giving him a small top-up prior to him going down for his nap. Once he has done a week of uninterrupted lunchtime naps, you can gradually cut back on the top-up until you have eliminated it altogether and he is back to having a full feed at 10.30am. However, should you find that your baby is more unsettled at the lunchtime nap without a top-up, there is no reason why you should not continue to offer it. The most important thing at this stage is that your baby sleeps well at the lunchtime nap.

- If your baby is waking up before 3am, refer to page 107 on how to implement a split late feed, which should help him sleep a longer spell in the night.

9

Weeks Six to Eight

Routine – six to eight weeks

Feed times	Nap times between 7am and 7pm
7am	9–9.45am
10.45am	11.45am/12 noon–2–2.30pm
2–2.30pm	4.30–5pm
5pm	6.15pm
10–10.30pm	Maximum daily sleep: 4 hours

Expressing times: 7.30am and 9.30pm

7am

- Baby should be awake, nappy changed and feeding no later than 7am.

- If he fed before 5am, he needs up to 15–20 minutes from the full breast. If he's still hungry, offer up to 10–15 minutes from the breast that you have expressed 30–60ml (1–2oz) from.

- If he fed at 6am, offer him up to 15–20 minutes from the second breast after expressing 30–60ml (1–2oz).

- Do not feed baby after 8am, as it will put him off his next feed.

- He can stay awake for up to two hours.

- Try to have breakfast no later than 8am while your baby has a kick on his play mat.

- Wash and dress baby, remembering to cream all his creases and dry skin.

8.50am

- Check baby's nappy and start winding down now.

9am

- Settle baby in his bed, half-swaddled, no later than 9am. He needs a nap of no longer than 45 minutes.

- Wash and sterilise bottles and expressing equipment.

9.45am

- Unswaddle baby so that he can wake up naturally.

10am

- Baby must be fully awake now, regardless of how long he slept.

- If baby had a full feed at 7am, he should last until nearer 10.45am for his next feed. If he fed earlier, followed by a top-up between 7am and 8am, he may need to start this feed slightly earlier.

- Encourage baby to have a good kick on his play mat.

10.45am

- Baby should be given up to 20–25 minutes from the breast he last fed on, then offered up to 10–15 minutes from the second breast, while you drink a large glass of water.

11.30am

- If baby was very alert and awake during the previous two hours, he may start to get tired by 11.30am and would need to be in bed by 11.45am.

11.45am

- Regardless of what baby has done earlier, he should now be winding down for his nap.

- Check the draw sheet and change his nappy.

- Settle baby in his bed, half- or fully swaddled, no later than 12 noon.

12 noon–2–2.30pm

- Baby needs a nap of no longer than two and a half hours from the time he went down.

- If he wakes up after 45 minutes, check the swaddle, but do not overstimulate him with lots of talking or eye contact.

- Allow 10–20 minutes for him to settle himself; if he is still unsettled, offer him half his 2pm feed and try to settle him back to sleep until 2pm.

- If he does not go back to sleep you will then need to give him a short catnap after his next feed so that he gets through happily until his late afternoon nap.

12 noon

- Wash and sterilise expressing equipment if you didn't do this earlier, then you should have lunch and a rest before the next feed.

2–2.30pm

- Baby must be awake and feeding no later than 2.30pm, regardless of how long he has slept.

- Unswaddle him and allow him to wake naturally. Change his nappy.

- Give him up to 15–20 minutes from the breast he last fed on. If he is still hungry, offer him up to 10–15 minutes from the other breast, while you drink a large glass of water.

- Do not feed baby after 3.15pm as it will put him off his next feed.

- If he had a broken lunchtime nap and didn't settle back to sleep, he will need to have a short catnap of 20 minutes fairly soon after his feed. He will then be ready for another nap around 4.30pm. By splitting the nap you will ensure that he doesn't sleep too much in the afternoon, which could result in him not settling well at 7pm.

- It is very important that he is fully awake now until 4.30pm, so he goes down well at 7pm; if he was very alert in the morning, he may be sleepier now. Do not overdress him, as extra warmth will make him drowsy.

- Lay baby on his play mat and encourage him to have a good kick.

4.15–4.30pm

- Change baby's nappy.

- This is a good time to take him for a walk to ensure that he naps well, and is refreshed for his next feed and bath.

- Baby should not sleep after 5pm if you want him to go down well at 7pm.

5pm

- Baby must be fully awake and feeding no later than 5pm.

- Give him up to 20 minutes from the breast he last fed on, while you drink a large glass of water.

- It is very important that he waits for the other breast until after his bath.

5.45pm

- If baby has been very wakeful during the day, or didn't nap well between 4.30pm and 5pm, he may need to start his bath and next feed early.

- Allow baby a good kick without his nappy, while you prepare things needed for his bath and bedtime.

6pm

- Baby must start his bath no later than 6pm, and be massaged and dressed by 6.15pm.

6.15pm

- Baby must be feeding no later than 6.15pm; this should be done in a quiet, dimly lit room with care taken to not over-stimulate him with lots of talking or eye contact.

- If he did not finish the first breast at 5pm, give him up to 5–10 minutes from it before putting him on the second breast.

- It is very important that baby is in bed two hours from when he last woke.

6.45–7pm

- Settle baby in his bed, half-swaddled, no later than 7pm.

8pm

- It is very important that you have a really good meal and a rest before the next feed or expressing.

9.30pm

- If you have chosen to replace the late feed with a bottle feed, then express from both breasts now.

10–10.30pm

- Turn up the lights fully and unswaddle baby so that he can wake up naturally. Allow at least 10 minutes before feeding to ensure that he is fully awake, so that he can feed well.

- Lay out things for the nappy change, plus a spare draw sheet, muslin and swaddle blanket in case they are needed in the middle of the night.

- Give baby up to 20 minutes from the breast he last fed on, or most of his bottle-feed, change his nappy and re-swaddle him.

- Dim the lights and, with no talking or eye contact, give him up to 20 minutes from the second breast or the remainder of the bottle-feed.

- It is important that your baby is awake for a full hour at this stage.

In the night

- Your baby should be starting to sleep longer in the night now. If you find that your baby is still waking up before 3am and not settling without a feed, you need to look at his daytime feeding and sleeping.

- Firstly, try to increase the late feed. If he is refusing to take more at the late feed, I recommend you try offering a split feed for several nights to encourage him to sleep longer. If you wake him at 9.45pm, offer him as much milk as he will take at 10pm, then keep him awake and offer a further top-up feed at 11.15pm. The combination of being awake longer and taking extra milk usually helps him to sleep a little longer. You may have to try this for several nights for it to work. If after several nights the situation has not improved, then it is best to go back to having your baby awake for a shorter period at the late feed.

- Some babies wake up at the same time every night through habit not hunger. If this is the case, you could try the core night method (see page 322) and then settling him with a cuddle and a dummy. If he settles within 20 minutes and then sleeps for another hour or so, it is worth trying this for a few nights to break the waking habit. However, if he wakes a second time in the night it is important to feed him as to offer a cuddle and the dummy a second time could create a habit of him waking twice a night. By feeding him the second time he wakes will encourage him to drop the feed at the first waking, and also ensure that he doesn't lose the ability to self-settle in the night. Obviously, if he doesn't settle within 20 minutes, it is best to feed him as the last thing you want is for him to be awake for a lengthy time in the night.

- If he wakes between 4–5am, give one breast, then start the 7am feed on the fuller breast. With formula-fed babies I would recommend that you offer him half of his normal 7am feed, then offer the second half plus an extra ounce (30ml) to top him up between 7.30–8am.

- If he wakes up at 6am give him one breast, then the second at 7.30am after expressing. With formula-fed babies it is best to offer him as much of his normal feed as he will take, then offer a top-up feed between 7.30–8am.

- Keep the lights low and do not overstimulate him with lots of talking or eye contact. Only change his nappy if absolutely necessary, or if he is too sleepy to take a full feed.

Changes to be made during the six-to eight-week routine

Sleeping

Most babies who weigh over 4kg (9lb) should be sleeping longer in the night now, provided they are getting most of their daily nutritional needs between 6–7am and 11pm. They should also be sleeping no more than four hours between 7am and 7pm.

Once he has lasted longer for several nights in a row, try not to feed your baby before his latest time again. The morning nap should be no more than 45 minutes, the lunchtime nap should be two and a quarter to two and a half hours – no longer – and the late afternoon nap should be no more than 30 minutes. He may catnap on and off during this nap and some babies cut out this nap altogether. Do not allow him to cut out this nap if he is not managing to stay awake until 7pm. If you want him to sleep until 7am, it is important that he goes to sleep nearer 7pm. Between six and eight weeks, you should ensure that your baby's morning nap is no longer than 45 minutes, as allowing longer than this could result in a shorter lunchtime nap. If you notice that your baby has already become more unsettled at lunchtime, despite offering a top-up prior to his nap, I would suggest cutting this nap to 30 minutes, even if it means bringing the time of the lunchtime nap forward slightly.

Lunchtime nap

From six weeks onwards, if your baby is sleeping the full 45 minutes in the morning, he should be woken after two and a quarter hours. If for some reason his morning nap was much shorter, then you could allow him two and a half hours.

- It is at around eight weeks that the lunchtime nap may sometimes go wrong: you may find that your baby wakes up 30–40 minutes after falling asleep and is unsettled. This is due to your baby taking on a more adult sleep cycle as he drifts from light sleep into a dream-like sleep (known as REM), then back into a deep sleep. While some babies only stir when they come into light sleep, others will wake up fully. If your baby has not learned to settle himself and is consistently assisted back to sleep, then a real problem could develop. If he is waking during his lunchtime nap (and you are already offering a top-up prior to settling him), allow him 10–20 minutes to see if he will resettle himself. If he is unable to return to sleep, or he becomes distressed at any point, go straight to him and offer him half of his 2pm feed (treat as a night feed) before returning him to his bed. If, even after this, he is still unsettled, just get him up for the afternoon.

- Obviously, if his lunchtime nap was cut short, he cannot make it through from 1pm to 4pm happily. I find the best way to deal with this is to allow a short cat nap after the 2–2.30pm feed, then a further cat nap after 4.30pm. This should stop him getting overtired and irritable and get things back on track so that he goes to sleep well at 7pm. See page 334 for more in-depth problem-solving.

- He should now be half-swaddled at the morning nap and 7pm sleep, and by the end of eight weeks also at the late feed and in the night.

Feeding

During growth spurts, if you have been expressing, you can reduce this by 30ml (1oz) to ensure that his needs are immediately met.

- If you have not expressed, you can still follow the feeding times from the routine for your baby's age, but you will have to top him up with a short breast-feed before his daytime naps. If you do this for a week or so, this should help increase your milk supply. A sign that this has happened is that your baby will sleep well at the naps, and not be so interested in the next feed. Once this happens you can gradually decrease the length of time that you top-up for, until you are back on your original feeding schedule.

- A formula-fed baby should have his feeds increased by 30ml (1oz) when he is regularly draining his bottle, starting with the morning feed. The late feed should only be increased if all the other feeds have been increased, and he is not going a longer spell in the night. Some babies will need to move to a medium-flow teat with three holes at this stage.

- Between the ages of six to eight weeks, a baby who is gaining weight steadily and weighs over 4kg (9lb) should manage to go a longer spell of around five to six hours in the night from his late feed, provided he is feeding well during the day and not sleeping more than the recommended amounts.

- If your baby is still waking between 2–3am, despite taking a good-sized feed, I would advise, if you are not already doing so, that you give a split feed at 10/11.15pm. The extra milk and time awake is often enough to help the baby sleep longer in the night. For this to work it is important that you start to wake your baby no later than 9.45pm, so that he is fully awake and feeding by 10pm. Allow him to drink as much of the feed as he would want, then allow him a good kick on the floor on his play mat. At 11pm you should then take him to the bedroom and change his nappy, then offer him a further feed. If you are formula-feeding, I would advise that you make a fresh feed up for the second feed.

- If your baby then wakes in the night, check that he has not kicked off his covers as this is another cause of night-time waking in babies of this age. See page 7 for advice on how to tuck your baby in securely. If he is securely tucked in but still waking, you should then try to settle him with a cuddle or a dummy (see core night method on page 322).

- If he refuses to settle, then you will have to feed him, but it would be advisable to refer to chapters 4 and 16 to check for possible reasons why he is not sleeping for longer in the night. If he does settle, he will probably wake up again at around 5am, at which time you can give him a full feed, followed by a top-up at 7.30–8am. This will help keep him on track with his feeding and sleeping pattern for the rest of the day.

- Keep increasing day feeds, not night feeds. Most babies are happy to wait longer after the 7am feed, so keep pushing this feed forward until your baby is feeding at 10.45am.

- During this stage, if your baby is taking a top-up at 7–8am instead of a full feed, he may not manage to get through to 10.45–11am for his next feed. You may need to give him half a feed at 10–10.15am, followed by a top-up just before he goes down for his lunchtime nap, to ensure that he does not wake up early from the nap. If your baby goes back to waking up earlier again, wait 10 minutes or so before going to him. If he will not settle himself back to sleep, try settling him with a cuddle or a dummy. If he doesn't settle back quickly, then you can try giving him half of his 2–2.30pm feed early and try again to settle him back to sleep. If this doesn't work it is easier just to get him up then offer a short catnap after the remainder of his 2–2.30pm feed, so that he gets through happily to his late afternoon nap.

10

Weeks Eight to Twelve

Routine – eight to twelve weeks

Feed times	Nap times between 7am and 7pm
7am	9–9.45am
10.45–11am	12–2–2.15pm
2–2.15pm	4.45–5pm
5pm	
6–6.15pm	
10–10.30pm	Maximum daily sleep: $3\frac{1}{2}$ hours

Expressing time: 9.30pm

7am

- Baby should be awake, nappy changed and feeding no later than 7am.

- He should be given up to 20 minutes from the first breast, then offered up to 10–15 minutes from the second breast.

- Do not feed baby after 7.45am, as it will put him off his next feed.

- He can stay awake for up to two hours.

- Try to have breakfast and a drink no later than 8am while baby has a kick on his play mat.

- Wash and dress baby, remembering to cream all his creases and dry skin.

8.50am

- Check baby's nappy and draw sheet.

9am

- Settle baby in his bed, half-swaddled, no later than 9am. He needs a nap of no longer than 45 minutes.
- Wash and sterilise bottles and expressing equipment.

9.45am

- Unswaddle baby so that he can wake up naturally.

10am

- Baby must be fully awake now, regardless of how long he slept.
- Encourage him to have a good kick on his play mat.

10.45–11am

- Baby should be given up to 20 minutes from the breast he last fed on, then offered up to 10–15 minutes from the second breast, while you drink a large glass of water.

11.45am

- Regardless of what baby has done earlier, he should now be winding down for his nap.
- Change his nappy and check the draw sheet.
- Settle baby in his bed, half-swaddled, no later than 12 noon.

12 noon–2/2.15pm

- Baby needs a nap of no longer than two and a quarter hours from the time he went down.

- If he wakes up after 45 minutes allow 10–20 minutes for him to resettle himself; if he is still unsettled, offer him half his 2pm feed and try to settle him back to sleep until 2–2.15pm.

- If he does not go back to sleep you will then need to give him a short cap nap after his next feed so that he gets through happily until his afternoon nap.

- Wash and sterilise bottles and expressing equipment if you didn't do this earlier, then you should have lunch and a rest before the next feed.

2–2.15pm

- Baby must be awake two and a quarter hours from the time he went down, regardless of how long he has slept and he must be feeding no later than 2.30pm.

- Unswaddle him and allow him to wake naturally. Change his nappy.

- Give him up to 20 minutes from the breast he last fed on. If he is still hungry offer him up to 10–15 minutes from the other breast, while you drink a large glass of water.

- Try not to feed baby after 3.15pm as it will put him off his next feed.

- If he had a broken lunchtime nap and didn't settle back to sleep, he will need to have a short cat-nap of 20 minutes fairly soon after his feed. He will then be ready for another nap around 4.30pm. By splitting the nap you will ensure that he doesn't sleep too much in the afternoon, which could result in him not settling well at 7pm.

- It is very important that he is fully awake now nearer 4.45pm, so he goes down well at 7pm.

4.15pm

- Change baby's nappy, and offer him a small drink of cool boiled water no later than 4.30pm.

- He may have a short nap between 4.45–5pm.

- Baby should not sleep after 5pm if you want him to go down well at 7pm.

5pm

- Baby should be fully awake and feeding no later than 5pm.

- Give him up to 15 minutes from the breast he last fed on, while you drink a large glass of water.

5.45pm

- If baby has been very wakeful during the day or didn't nap well between 4.45–5pm, he may need to start his bath and next feed early.

- Allow baby a good kick without his nappy, while you prepare things needed for his bath and bedtime.

6pm

- Baby must start his bath no later than 6pm, and be massaged and dressed by 6.15pm.

6.15pm

- Baby must be feeding no later than 6.15pm; this should be done in a quiet, dimly lit room with care taken not to over-stimulate him with lots of talking or eye contact.

- If he did not finish the first breast at 5pm, give him up to 5–10 minutes from it before putting him on the second breast. Allow up to 20 minutes from the second breast.

- It is very important that baby is in bed two hours from when he last woke.

7pm

- Settle baby in his bed, half-swaddled, no later than 7pm.

8pm

- It is very important that you have a really good meal and a rest before the next feed or expressing.

9.30pm

- If you have chosen to replace the late feed with a bottle feed, then express from both breasts now.

10–10.30pm

- Turn up the lights fully and unswaddle baby so that he can wake up naturally. Allow at least 10 minutes before feeding to ensure that he is fully awake, so that he can feed well.

- Lay out things for the nappy change, plus a spare draw sheet, muslin and swaddle blanket in case they are needed in the middle of the night.

- Give baby up to 20 minutes from the first breast or most of his bottle-feed, change his nappy and re-swaddle him using a half swaddle.

- Dim the lights and, with no talking or eye contact, give him up to 20 minutes from the second breast or the remainder of the bottle-feed.

In the night

- If your baby is feeding before 5am, feeding well and losing interest in his 7am feed, it would be worth trying the core night method (see page 322). Remember, the aim is to get him to take all his daily requirements between 6–7am and 11pm.

- If he wakes up at 5am, give him one breast and, if needed, 5–10 minutes from the second breast. With formula-fed babies I would recommend that you offer him half of his normal 7am feed, and then offer the second half plus an extra ounce (30ml) at 7am–8am.

- If he wakes up at 6am, give him one breast, then the second at 7.30am. With formula-fed babies, give him as much of his normal feed as he will take, then offer a top-up feed at 7.30am/8am.

- Keep the lights low and do not overstimulate him with lots of talking or eye contact. Only change his nappy if absolutely necessary or if he is too sleepy to take a full feed.

Changes to be made during the eight-to twelve-week routine

Sleeping

Many babies who are nearer 5.4kg (12lb) in weight can manage to go through the night from the late feed at this age, provided they are taking all their daily nutritional needs between 6–7am and 11pm. They should also be sleeping no more than three and a half hours between 7am and 7pm. A totally breast-fed baby may still be waking up once in the night, hopefully nearer 6–7am.

- Gradually cut back your baby's daily nap time by a further 30 minutes, to a total of three and a half hours. The morning nap should be no more than 45 minutes if you want him to sleep well at the lunch time nap.

- The lunchtime nap should be no more than two and a quarter hours. It is around this stage that the lunchtime nap can sometimes go wrong. The baby comes into a light sleep usually 30–45 minutes after he has gone to sleep. Some babies will wake up fully and it is important that they learn how to settle themselves back to sleep to avoid the wrong sleep associations. For more details on this problem, refer to page 339. Most babies have cut out their late afternoon nap by now. If your baby hasn't, do not allow him to sleep for more than 15 minutes, unless for some reason the lunchtime nap has gone wrong and then it would be slightly longer.

- All babies should only be half-swaddled and particular attention should be paid when tucking the baby in. One reason many babies of this age still wake up in the night is because they kick off the covers and move around the cot. If this is happening with your baby, I would advise that you purchase a 0.5 tog light summer-weight sleeping bag. They are so lightweight that you can still use a sheet to tuck your baby in, without the worry of overheating. (See pages 5–8 for further details on cots and bedding.)

Feeding

Your baby should be well established on five feeds a day now. If he is totally breast-fed and has started waking up earlier in the morning, it may be worth trying a top-up from a bottle of either expressed or formula milk after the late feed. If he is sleeping regularly until 7am, gradually bring the late feed forward by five minutes every three nights until he is feeding at 10pm. As long as he continues to sleep through to 7am and takes a full feed, you can keep pushing the 10.45am feed forward until he is feeding at 11am.

- Once your baby has slept through the night for two weeks, the 5pm feed can be dropped if your baby shows signs of losing interest in it. I would not recommend dropping the split feed until this happens, as a larger feed at 6.15pm could result in your baby taking even less at the last feed, resulting in an earlier waking time.

- With many of the babies that I cared for, I kept giving them a split feed until solids were introduced to ensure that they were getting enough milk during the day. Once you eliminate the 5pm feed and your baby is taking a full feed after his bath, he could cut down dramatically on his last feed of the day, which could result in an early waking. If this happens, it is advisable to reintroduce a split feed at 5–6.15pm until your baby is fully established on solids and sleeping through to nearer 7am.

- If you are breast-feeding and considering introducing a further bottle-feed, the best time to introduce it is at the 11am feed. Gradually reduce the time on the breast by two or three minutes each day and top up with formula.

By the end of the first week, if your baby is taking a bottle-feed of 150–180ml (5–6oz), you should be able to drop the breast-feed easily without the risk of serious engorgement. Bottle-fed babies should continue to have their 7am, 11am and 6.15pm feeds increased first during the next growth spurt at around nine weeks. Increase the bottle-feed to suit your baby's needs.

Moving on to the three- to four-month routine

As long as you are not exceeding your baby's daytime sleep, and he is following the eight- to twelve-week routine at night, then you can move on to the next routine. However if, despite following all the advice, your baby is not sleeping as long in the night as the routine suggests, stick with this routine and try to improve the night sleeping. It might be worth delaying the late feed until nearer midnight, or dropping it altogether for a short period, to try to establish a longer period of sleep from 7pm onwards. Once a longer period of sleep becomes established, the late feed can be reinstated, and hopefully the baby's longer spell of sleep will then happen between 11pm and 6–7am. The best way to reinstate the feed is to gradually bring it back from midnight by ten minutes every two or three nights until he is back to feeding at 10–10.30pm, and hopefully the baby's longer spell will happen between 11pm and 6–7am. Once this happens, you can then move on to the three-to four-month routine.

11

Months Three to Four

Routine – three to four months

Feed times	Nap times between 7am and 7pm
7am	9–9.45am
11am	12–2–2.15 pm
2.15–2.30pm	
5pm	
6–6.15pm	
10–10.30pm	Maximum daily sleep: 3 hours
Expressing time: 9.30pm	

7am

- Baby should be awake, nappy changed and feeding no later than 7am.

- He should be given a full feed from both breasts or a full bottle-feed.

By this stage, most babies reduce the amount of time they need to feed on the breast. Be guided by your baby. If he is going happily from one feed to the next then he is likely to be getting enough milk.

- He can stay awake for around two hours.

8am

- Baby should be encouraged to have a good kick on his play mat while you have breakfast.

- Wash and dress baby, remembering to cream all his creases and dry skin.

9am

- Settle baby in his bed, half-swaddled, no later than 9am. He needs a nap of no longer than 45 minutes.

- Wash and sterilise bottles and expressing equipment.

9.45am

- Unswaddle baby so that he can wake up naturally.

10am

- Baby must be fully awake now, regardless of how long he slept.

- Encourage him to have a good kick on his play mat or take him on an outing.

11am

- Baby should be given a feed from both breasts or a full bottle-feed.

11.50am

- Check the draw sheet and change his nappy.

- Settle baby, half-swaddled, no later than 12 noon.

12 noon–2–2.15pm

- Baby needs a nap of no longer than two and a quarter hours from the time he went down.

- Wash and sterilise bottles and expressing equipment if you didn't do this earlier, then you should have lunch and a rest before the next feed.

2–2.15pm

- Regardless of how long he has slept baby should be awake and feeding no later than 2.30pm.

- Unswaddle him and allow him to wake naturally. Change his nappy.

- He should be given a feed from both breasts or a bottle-feed.

- Try not to feed baby after 3.15pm as it will put him off his next feed.

- If he had a broken lunchtime nap and didn't settle back to sleep, he will need to have a short cat-nap of 20 minutes fairly soon after his feed. He will then be ready for another nap around 4.30pm. By splitting the nap you will ensure that he doesn't sleep too much in the afternoon, which could result in him not settling well at 7pm.

- If he has slept well at both naps, he should manage to get through the rest of the afternoon without a further sleep.

4–4.15pm

- Change baby's nappy and offer him a drink of cool boiled water no later than 4.30pm.

- If he did not sleep so well at lunchtime, he may need a short nap sometime between now and 5pm.

- Baby should not sleep after 5pm if you want him to go down well at 7pm.

5pm

- Give him up to 15 minutes from the breast he last fed on, or half a bottle-feed.

5.45pm

- Allow baby a good kick without his nappy, while you prepare things needed for his bath and bedtime.

6pm

- Baby must start his bath no later than 6pm, and be massaged and dressed by 6.15pm.

6.15pm

- Baby must be feeding no later than 6.15pm.

- If he did not finish the first breast at 5pm, give him up to 5–10 minutes from it before putting him on the second breast. Allow him up to 20 minutes from the second breast or a bottle-feed.

- A bottle-fed baby should be offered half a bottle feed, plus an extra ounce.

- Dim the lights and sit baby in his chair for 10 minutes while you tidy up.

7pm

- Settle baby in his bed, half-swaddled, no later than 7pm.

8pm

- It is very important that you have a really good meal and a rest before the next feed or expressing.

9.30pm

- If you have chosen to replace the late feed with a bottle feed, then express from both breasts now.

10–10.30pm

- Turn up the lights and unswaddle baby so that he can wake up naturally.

- Give him most of his breast-feed or bottle-feed, change his nappy and half-swaddle him.

- Dim the lights and, with no talking or eye contact, give him the remainder of his feed.

Changes to be made during the three- to four-month routine

Sleeping

If you have structured the milk feeds and nap times according to the routine, your baby should manage to sleep through the night from the late feed to nearer 6–7am in the morning. If he shows signs of starting to wake up earlier, assume that it may be due to hunger. Increase his late feed and, if need be, go back to offering a split feed at this time. By the time he reaches four months try to aim for a maximum daily sleep total of three hours between 7am and 7pm. Some babies may need less sleep than this, and you may have to look at cutting his total daytime sleep back to around two and a half hours, with a 30-minute nap in the morning, and a two-hour nap at lunchtime.

- If your baby is following the routine well, he will have cut right back on his late afternoon nap and some days may manage to get through the afternoon without the nap, but may need to go to bed 5–10 minutes earlier on those days.

- Should your baby have slept less than two hours at lunchtime, he should certainly be encouraged to have a short nap of no longer than 15–30 minutes between 4–5pm depending on how he slept at lunchtime otherwise he may become so overtired at bedtime that he doesn't settle to sleep easily.

- Between three and four months, the time that your baby is awake at the late feed should be gradually reduced to 30 minutes, provided he has been sleeping through regularly to 7am, for at least two weeks. This should be very quiet and treated like a middle-of-the-night feed. Bring it forward by 10 minutes every three nights until it becomes a very quick, sleepy feed at 10pm.

- If, despite following all the advice I have given about dealing with night waking, your baby is still waking, then I would recommend that for several days you could try leaving your baby until 11.45pm and then giving him a dream feed to see if that will help him sleep later.

- However, if your baby is still waking up between 5–6am after several days, it would be advisable to try and keep him awake for at least an hour at the late feed, following the suggestions for the split feed.

- Even if he is not getting out of his half-swaddle, if you have not already done so, I would suggest that now is a good time to get him used to a 100 per cent cotton, very lightweight sleeping bag; it is important that you purchase a 0.5 tog sleeping bag to avoid the risk of overheating. He will still need to be tucked in firmly, with one sheet, and perhaps one blanket, depending on the room temperature, so that he cannot kick off his covers (see page 6 for advice on how to make up the cot).

Feeding

Between three to four months, if your baby has slept through the night until 7am for at least two weeks, you should try to ensure that any extra milk needed during growth spurts is increased at daytime feeds to prevent him backtracking on his night-time waking.

- If your baby is totally breast-fed and is still waking up in the night, despite being topped up with expressed milk at the late feed, it could be that he will need an increased feed at this time. If you are unable to express extra milk earlier in the day, some mothers find that topping up with a small amount of formula at this feed helps. You should discuss this with your health visitor. If your baby is formula-fed 210–240ml (7–8oz) four times a day, he may only need a small feed of 120–180ml (4–6oz) at the late feed. However, if your baby is not sleeping through the night at this age, it may be because he needs a little extra at this feed. Even if it means he cuts back on his morning feed, I would suggest offering him a full feed of 210–240ml (7–8oz) for several nights to see if that will help him sleep for longer in the night.

- If you find that more milk at the late feed helps your baby sleep through to 7am, but he then cuts down his 7am feed, I would advise that it is better for a short time to accept this and have him sleeping through, than giving too small a feed at the late feed. When he takes a smaller feed at 7am, you will need to bring his 11am feed forward with a top up just before the lunch time nap.

- There are some babies who simply refuse the late feed at three to four months. However, if you find that he starts to wake earlier again and will not settle back to sleep within 10 minutes or so, you would have to assume that it could be hunger and feed him. You may then have to consider reintroducing the late feed until he is weaned and established on solids.

- If you find that your baby keeps on waking before 4–5am in the night, and will not settle without feeding, keep a very detailed diary listing exact times and amounts of feeding and times of daytime naps, to try to determine whether the waking is habit or actual hunger.

- Whether you are breast-feeding or bottle-feeding, if your baby's weight gain is good and you are convinced he is waking up from habit, try waiting 15–20 minutes before going to him. Some babies will actually settle themselves back to sleep. A baby of this age may still be waking up in the night because he is getting out of his covers. Tuck him in securely (see page 7).

- If your baby is formula-fed and is taking 995–1130ml (35–40oz) of formula between 7am and 11pm, he should not really need to feed in the night. However, some very big babies who weigh over 6.8kg (15lb) at this stage may still need to feed between 5–6am, followed by a top-up at 7–7.30am until they reach six months and are weaned.

- A totally breast-fed baby may need to feed at around 5–6am as he may not be getting enough to eat at the last feed. Regardless of whether they are breast- or bottle-fed, a good indicator of whether your baby is ready to drop the night feed is how he takes his top-up at 7–7.30am. If he takes it greedily, he is probably genuinely hungry at 5–6am. If he fusses and frets and refuses the top-up, I would assume the early wake-up was more habit than hunger and try to settle him back with a cuddle.

- If your baby continues to sleep through to 7am once his waking time at the late feed has been reduced to 30 minutes, plus he is cutting back on his 7am feed, start very slowly reducing the amount he is drinking at the late feed. Only continue with this if he is sleeping well until 7am. However, I would not advise dropping this feed altogether until he is between six and seven months and solids have been established. If you abandon the late feed before solids are introduced, and your baby goes through a growth spurt, you may find that you have to go back to feeding him in the middle of the night again.

- If your baby is exclusively breast-fed and is over 6.3kg (14lb) in weight, you may find that during growth spurts you have to go back to feeding him in the middle of the night anyway, until solids are introduced. If you feel that your milk supply is low, follow the plan for increasing milk supply on page 313.

- Some babies start to totally refuse the late feed at this age, but are not able to sleep twelve hours without the fifth feed. If this happens you will have to accept that your baby may need to feed between 4–6am until solids are introduced. If he is waking at this time, do not be tempted to try and push him through without a feed, as this could lead to a habit of him being awake on and off, which could lead to a long-term early morning waking problem. If he is going from 7pm to between 4–6am, he is still doing really well sleeping such a long time, therefore when he wakes it is better to feed him and get him back to sleep quickly.

12

Months Four to Six

Routine – four to six months

Feed times	Nap times between 7am and 7pm
7am	9–9.45am
11am	12–2.15 pm
2.15–2.30pm	
6–6.15pm	
10pm	Maximum daily sleep: 3 hours

Expressing time: 9.30pm

7am

- Baby should be awake, nappy changed and feeding no later than 7am.

- He should be given a full feed from both breasts or a full bottle-feed.

- He can stay awake for around two hours.

8am

- Baby should be encouraged to have a good kick on his mat or play with some age appropriate toys for 20–30 minutes while you have breakfast.

- Wash and dress baby, remembering to cream all his creases and dry skin.

9–9.15am

- Settle baby in his sleeping bag, securely tucked in, no later than 9.15am. He needs a nap of 30–45 minutes.

9.45am

- Untuck him so that he can wake up naturally.

10am

- Baby must be fully awake now, regardless of how long he slept.
- Encourage him to have a good kick on his play mat or take him on an outing.

11am

- Baby should be given a feed from both breasts or a full bottle-feed before being offered solids, if you have been advised to wean early (see page 257).
- Encourage him to sit in his chair while you clear away the lunch things.

11.50am

- Check the draw sheet and change his nappy.
- Settle baby in his sleeping bag, securely tucked in, no later than 12 noon.

12–12.15pm

- Baby needs a nap of no longer than two and a quarter hours from the time he went down.

2–2.15pm

- Regardless of how long he has slept, baby should be awake and feeding no later than 2.30pm.

- Untuck baby and allow him to wake naturally. Change his nappy.

- He should be given a feed from both breasts or a bottle-feed.

- Do not feed baby after 3.15pm as it will put him off his next feed.

- If he has slept well at both naps, he should manage to get through the rest of the afternoon without a further sleep.

4.15pm

- If he did not sleep so well at lunchtime, he may need a short nap sometime between now and 5pm.

- Baby should not sleep after 5pm if you want him to go down well at 7pm.

5pm

- Some babies are happy to wait until after the bath for his feed. If not, offer him up to 10–15 minutes from the breast he last fed on, or half a bottle-feed.

- If you have been advised to wean your baby early, I would recommend that you offer him half of his milk feed before offering him the solids so that his milk intake does not decrease too rapidly.

5.30pm

- Allow baby a good kick without his nappy, while you prepare things needed for his bath and bedtime.

5.45pm

- Baby must start his bath no later than 5.45pm, and be massaged and dressed between 6–6.15pm.

6–6.15pm

- Baby should start his feed between 6–6.15pm, depending on how tired he is.

- Babies who have been fed solids will probably not be ready for their milk feed until nearer 6.15–6.30pm.

- He should be given a full feed from both breasts or have a full bottle-feed. If he fed at 5pm but did not finish the first breast, give him up to 5–10 minutes from it before putting him on the second breast. Allow him up to 20 minutes from the second breast or a bottle-feed.

- A bottle fed baby should be offered half a bottle, plus an extra ounce.

- Dim the lights and sit baby in his chair for 10 minutes while you tidy up.

7pm

- Settle baby in his sleeping bag, securely tucked in, no later than 7pm.

- It is very important that you have a really good meal and a rest before the next feed or expressing.

9.30pm

- If you have chosen to replace the late feed with a bottle feed, then express from both breasts now.

10pm

- Turn up the lights and wake baby enough to feed.

- Remove his sleeping bag, give him most of the feed, change his nappy and then replace his sleeping bag.

- Dim the lights and, with no talking or eye contact, give him the remainder of the feed. If he does not want the remainder, do not force it; he could start to cut back on this feed now.

- This feed should take no longer than 30 minutes.

- Tuck baby in securely with a thin sheet.

Changes to be made during the four-to six-month routine

Sleeping

Between four and six months, most babies can manage to sleep from the late feed until 6–7am in the morning, provided they are taking four to five full milk feeds a day, and not sleeping more than three hours between 7am and 7pm. Some breast-fed babies may still need a feed around 5am if there are not taking a big enough feed at the late feed.

- If your baby is still waking in the night and you are confident that it is not due to hunger, I would advise trying the 'core night method', as described on page 322. If this does not work, it could be that he is a baby who needs less sleep, and I would suggest gradually cutting back on his daytime sleep by a couple of minutes every few days until you've reduced by 10–15 minutes a day.

- If after a couple of weeks this has not improved things, then I would suggest dropping the late feed to see how long he will sleep. The time he wakes up will help you decide whether to continue with the late feed. For example, if he sleeps between 3–5am, then feeds and settles back to sleep until 7am, he will at least be sleeping one longer spell between 7pm and 7am, and this would be preferable to him waking and feeding at both the late feed and 5am.

- However, if you drop the feed and he wakes at something like 1am and 5am, then it would make sense to continue with the late feed so that he doesn't wake and feed twice between midnight and 5am.

- If your baby weighs over 6.8kg (15lb) genuine hunger could be the cause of night waking, particularly if he is fully breast-fed. If this is the case, then you may have to accept that he will need a breast-feed in the night until he is established on solids at six months.

- If you feel that he is showing signs that he is ready to be weaned, consult your health visitor or GP for advice as to whether he should begin earlier than the recommended six months. If you decide to continue to feed him in the middle of the night, it is crucial to ensure that feeds are given quickly and quietly and that he settles back to sleep quickly and sleeps soundly until 7am.

- If you have not already introduced a sleeping bag, it would be advisable to do so at this stage. If you leave it any later, he may be unhappy about being put into one.

- Until your baby is able to crawl and manoeuvre himself around the cot, he still needs to sleep on his back and be tucked in firmly. In very hot weather he can be put into a 0.5 tog sleeping bag, with just a nappy on, and tucked in with a very thin cotton sheet. It is important that at least 15cm (6in) of the sheet is tucked under the mattress so that your baby cannot kick it off.

- Once your baby starts to roll on to his tummy, it is essential that you remove the sheet so that he does not get caught up in it. You may find that for a short period you will have to go in to him in the middle of the night if he gets stuck in a corner or a difficult position. During this stage of development, it is important that you spend time during the day teaching him to roll from his back to his front and front to back.

- If he is not sleeping the full two hours at lunchtime, try pushing his morning nap a little later and gradually reduce it by 10–15 minutes. Then bring the 11am feed forward to 10.30am. Top him up with some milk just before he goes down for his lunchtime nap.

Feeding

I recommend that you still continue to feed your baby at the late feed until solids are well established. The current guidelines are that solids should now be introduced at six months, rather than at four months as previously recommended. As your baby will continue to go through growth spurts between four and six months, his nutritional needs will still need to be met. In my experience this can rarely be done on four milk feeds a day.

- If you decide to drop the late feed and he starts to wake earlier and not settle back to sleep quickly, then you should assume that it is hunger and feed him. It would then be worth considering reintroducing the late feed until solids are established.

- If you find that he refuses a late feed, but wakes up at 5am hungry, then you should feed him and settle him back to sleep until 7am, then offer him a top-up feed before 8am. If this happens, you may then have to feed him earlier, between 10–10.30am, but then I would suggest that you offer him a further top-up before he goes down for his lunchtime nap, to ensure that he does sleep well.

- During growth spurts, you may find that your baby is not content on five feeds a day. If this is the case, you may have to offer a split feed (see page 173) in the morning and reintroduce the 5pm feed if you had previously dropped it. If your baby becomes very discontented between feeds, despite being offered extra milk, and you think that he is showing signs of needing to be weaned, then it is important to discuss this with your health visitor or GP.

- If weaning your baby before six months is recommended, then it is important to introduce solids very carefully. Solids should only be seen as tasters at this stage and given in addition to milk; they should not be a replacement for milk feeds (see page 257). To ensure this does not happen always make sure that your baby takes all of his milk feed first.

- Start off with a small amount of baby rice mixed with either breast milk or formula milk after the 11am feed. Once he is taking this you can then transfer the rice to after he has had a milk feed at 5pm in the evening, then start to introduce some of the first weaning foods recommended on page 265–6 after the 11am feed.

- When introducing solids in the evening, offer half a milk feed at 5pm, followed by the solids, then after the bath offer him another half milk feed.

- Over the next two months gradually decrease the 5pm milk feed and increase solids. Then offer your baby a full milk feed after the bath.

- If you are formula-feeding, it is advisable to make up two separate bottles to ensure that the milk is fresh. Once solids are introduced at this feed, and as they increase, your baby should automatically cut back on his late feed.

- Once he is down to taking only a very short breast-feed or just a couple of ounces (60ml) of formula at the late feed, and continuing to sleep well through to 7am, you should be able to drop the late feed without risking that he will wake earlier in the morning.

- A breast-fed baby who has reached five months, is weaned, and is now starting to wake up before 10pm, may not be getting enough milk at the bedtime feed. Try offering a top-up of expressed milk or formula after baby has been fed from both breasts.

- A baby who is not weaned would more than likely need to continue to have a split milk feed at 5–6.15pm until solids are introduced. For more information on early weaning see page 257.

- A full milk feed for a bottle fed baby is 240ml (8oz). When doing split feeds, because of the space between them, it is fine to offer an extra ounce. For example you could split the feed by offering 150ml (5oz) and then 120ml (4oz) or vice versa.

13

Months Six to Nine

Once your baby reaches six months, you can get him used to sleeping in his own room. Because he will have been used to always having people around him during nap times and in the evening, it is best to do this gradually. Start off with settling him at either the morning or lunchtime nap in his own room. Once he is sleeping well at either of these times, you can then move on to settling him in his own room from 7pm. As your baby will not have been used to sleeping in the dark for daytime naps, I would suggest that you allow him a small night light for naps and at bedtime, until he is used to sleeping in his own room. Gradually phase this out once he is settling and sleeping well at these times.

Routine – six to nine months

Feed times	Nap times between 7am and 7pm
7am	9.15–9.30–10am
11.30am	12.30–2.30pm
2.30pm	
5pm	
6.30pm	Maximum daily sleep: $2\frac{1}{2}$–$2\frac{3}{4}$ hours

7am

- Baby should be awake, nappy changed and feeding no later than 7am.

- He should be given most of his breast feed or bottle feed, followed by breakfast solids, once weaning is established. Finish off with the remainder of his milk feed. Try to eat breakfast at the same time as your baby, as this will help encourage good eating habits from an early age.

- He can stay awake for two to two and a half hours.

8am

- Baby should be encouraged to play with age appropriate toys whilst you deal with any urgent household chores.

- Wash and dress baby, remembering to cream all his creases and dry skin.

9.15–9.30am

- Close the curtains and settle baby in his sleeping bag, in the dark with the door shut, no later than 9.30am. He needs a nap of 30–45 minutes.

9.55am

- Open the curtains and undo his sleeping bag so that he can wake up naturally.

- Baby must be fully awake by 10am, regardless of how long he slept.

- Encourage lots of physical activity, either at home or at an organised play group.

11.30am

- By seven months baby should be given most of his solids before being offered a drink of water from a beaker, then alternate between solids and a drink.

- Encourage him to sit in his chair with some finger foods (see page 274), while you have lunch.

- Keep pushing the time of your baby's lunch forward until it is nearer midday.

- Until your baby is drinking 60–90ml (2–3oz) of other fluids with his lunch, you can continue to offer him a small milk feed just prior to his lunch time nap.

12.20pm

- Check the draw sheet and change his nappy.

- Close the curtains and settle baby, in his sleeping bag, in the dark with the door shut, no later than 12.30pm.

12.30–2.30pm

- Baby needs a nap of no longer than two hours from the time he went down.

2.30pm

- Baby must be awake and feeding no later than 2.30pm, regardless of how long he has slept.

- If he has had a small milk feed prior to his lunch time nap, this feed will probably be much smaller.

- Open the curtains and undo his sleeping bag so that he can wake up naturally. Change his nappy.

- He should be given a feed from both breasts and bottle-fed babies should have their feed from a beaker.

- Do not feed baby after 3.15pm as it will put him off his next feed.

4.15pm

- Change baby's nappy.

5pm

- Baby should be given most of his solids before being offered a small drink of water from a beaker. It is important that he still has a good milk feed at bedtime, so keep this drink to a minimum.

6pm

- He must start his bath no later than 6pm, and be massaged and dressed by 6.30pm.

6.30pm

- Baby must be feeding no later than 6.30pm. He should be given a feed from both breasts or a full bottle-feed.

- Dim the lights and read him a story.

7pm

- Settle baby in his sleeping bag, in the dark with the door shut, no later than 7pm.

Changes to be made during the six- to nine-month routine

Sleeping

Once your baby is established on three meals a day, he should manage to sleep from around 7pm to 7am. If you have followed the most recent guidelines on weaning and started weaning your baby on to solids at six months, he may need a small late feed until he is nearer seven months until solids are well established. If you were advised to wean him before six months and solids were well established when he reached six months, you should be able to drop the late feed sooner.

- Once he reaches six months you should gradually push the morning nap forward to 9.30am. This will encourage him to go down for his lunchtime nap nearer to 12.30pm. This is important once solids are established and he is having three proper meals a day, with lunch coming around 11.45am–12 noon.

- Some babies are happy to sleep later in the morning once they are established on three solid meals a day. If your baby sleeps until nearer 8am, he will not need a morning nap, but may not manage to get through until 12.30pm for his lunchtime nap; therefore, he may need to have lunch around 11.30am so he can go down at 12.15pm for his lunchtime nap (see page 347).

- Between six and nine months, if he has not already done so, your baby will start to roll on to his tummy. When this happens, it is important to remove the sheet and blanket to avoid him getting into a tangle with them. In the winter months, the lightweight sleeping bag will need to be replaced with a warmer one to make up for the loss of blankets. Until he can manage to roll from his back to his front and back again, you will find that for a short spell you will have to help him return to sleeping on his back. During the day ensure that you encourage lots of practice of rolling both ways, so that any sleep disruptions are kept to a minimum.

- If you are going back to work and your baby starts going to nursery, you may find that in the early days he does not sleep as long at the lunchtime nap. This can mean having to deal with a very tired and grumpy baby who is ready to sleep long before his normal bedtime. Depending on how long your journey takes from nursery to your home, the problem can usually be resolved if he has a short catnap on the way home. If the car journey is very short, you may have to consider driving round for a little bit longer to enable your baby to have a short nap. Fortunately, most babies will start to fall into a better sleep routine after a few weeks, but it is important to stress to your nursery that you want your baby to have his longer sleep after lunch, rather than in the morning, other-wise the problem could continue.

Feeding

If you have waited until six months to introduce solids, it is important that you work through the different foods fairly quickly and keep increasing the amounts every couple of days or when your baby shows signs of wanting more. Start off by introducing baby rice after the 11am feed (see page 265), and then every couple of days introduce a new food, from the first-stage foods. Once your baby is taking a reasonable amount of solids at lunch and teatime, you can introduce solids at breakfast.

- Between six and seven months his 11am milk feed will gradu-ally be reduced as his solids increase and once protein is introduced it can be dropped altogether and replaced with a drink of water from a beaker. However, if you baby only takes a small amount of water, he may need to have a small top-up milk feed prior to his lunchtime nap, until he is used to taking a larger amount of water.

- If you were advised to wean your baby early, you will probably have worked your way through the list of first-stage weaning foods (see page 265) by the time he reaches six months. Once he is taking around six tablespoonfuls of mixed vegetables at lunchtime, you can then introduce the second-stage foods, which include protein. For details of how to introduce protein, see page 268. For more information on the first and second stages of weaning see pages 264–279.

- By the end of six months, your baby will probably be ready to sit in a high chair for his meals. Always ensure that he is properly strapped in and never left unattended.

- It is important that you introduce your baby to a beaker at lunchtime between the ages of six and seven months, and that you start to use the tier system of feeding at lunchtime. Once your baby is only taking a couple of ounces (60ml) of milk at lunchtime, replace it with a drink of water from a beaker. If you find that your baby starts to wake up earlier from his lunch time nap, I would recommend offering him a small top-up milk feed just prior to his lunch time nap. This may mean that he cuts down on his 2.30pm feed, but this is preferable to him cutting back on his lunch time sleep.

- Once the lunchtime milk is dropped, he may need to increase the 2.30pm feed. However, if you notice that he is cutting back too much on his bedtime feed, continue to keep this feed smaller. This feed should be given from a beaker at this age.

- Between six and seven months, milk prior to the solids at tea time should be dropped and your baby should go straight into solids at 5pm, with only a small drink of water from a beaker. He would then have a full milk feed around 6.30pm.

- Babies who are attending nursery will usually be given their tea around 3.30–4pm. Obviously you cannot expect your baby to go from that time right through to the morning without any further solid food, so you will have to offer him something when you get home. If he has had a full tea at nursery, he will not be hungry enough for another full meal, so offer him something like a vegetable bake, or some pasta and vegetable sauce, or even a bowl of cereal, but not so much that it puts him off his bedtime milk feed. However, if he has only had a small snack mid-afternoon at nursery, he will need a proper tea, but he may not eat quite as much as the days when he is at home and he has not had such a big mid-afternoon snack.

- By nine months, if your baby is formula-fed, he should be drinking all of his water and most of his milk feeds from a beaker.

- It is really important to begin to clean your baby's teeth as soon as the first one appears. At this stage you will probably find it easiest to use a small piece of clean gauze wrapped around your finger, along with a small amount of special baby toothpaste, which can be massaged all around the baby's gums and teeth. Later, when more teeth have appeared, you can move on to a soft baby toothbrush for cleaning.

- If your baby is not cutting down on his late feed once solids are established, it may be that he is not getting the right quantities of solids for his age or weight, or is not taking a full milk feed at 6.30pm. Breast-fed babies may need a small top up after this feed and bottle-fed babies should be taking 210–240ml (7–8oz). Keep a diary of all food and milk consumed over a period of four days to help pinpoint why he is not cutting out that last feed.

- If you are confident that he is getting the right amounts and is taking the late feed from habit rather than genuine hunger, I would suggest that you gradually start to reduce it. If you reduce it by an ounce every three to four days, provided he does not start to wake up early, you should continue to do this until he is taking only a couple of ounces (60ml). Once he is taking a couple of ounces, you can then drop it altogether and he can then sleep through from 7pm to 7am.

14

Months Nine to Twelve

Routine – nine to twelve months

Feed times	Nap times between 7am and 7pm
7am	9.30–10am
11.45am–12 noon	12.30–2.30 pm
2.30pm	
5pm	
6.30pm	Maximum daily sleep: 2–2½ hours

7am

- Baby should be awake, nappy changed and feeding no later than 7am.

- He should be given most of his breast feed or bottle feed, followed by breakfast solids, once weaning is established. Finish off with the remainder of his milk feed. Try to eat breakfast at the same time as your baby, as this will help encourage good eating habits from an early age.

- He can stay awake for at least two and a half hours.

8am

- Baby should be encouraged to play with age-appropriate toys.

- Wash and dress baby, remembering to cream all his creases and dry skin.

9.30am

- Close the curtains and settle baby in his sleeping bag, in the dark with the door shut, at around 9.30am. He needs a nap of 15–30 minutes.

9.55am

- Open the curtains and undo his sleeping bag so that he can wake up naturally.

- Baby must be fully awake by 10am, regardless of how long he slept.

- Encourage lots of physical activity, either at home or at an organised play group.

11.45am–12 noon

- Baby should be given most of his solids before being offered a drink of water or well-diluted juice from a beaker, then alternate between solids and a drink.

- Encourage him to sit in his chair with some finger foods, while you have lunch.

12.20pm

- Check the draw sheet and change his nappy.

- Close the curtains and settle baby in his sleeping bag, in the dark with the door shut, no later than 12.30pm.

- He needs a nap of no longer than two hours from the time he went down.

- If your baby is falling asleep for his morning nap much later than 10.30am, it would be wise to allow no more than 10-15 minutes so that he still goes down well for his lunch time nap at 12.30pm. If he sleeps much longer than this, you may find he is not ready for his lunch time nap until nearer 1pm. If this happens I would reduce the lunch time nap to 1 hour and 45 minutes if you want him to settle well at 7pm. If you give him the full two hours you may find that he will not be ready for bed until nearer 7.30pm.

2.30pm

- If he slept at 12.30pm he should be awake no later than 2.30pm, if you want him to be ready for bed at 7pm.

- If he had a late morning nap and went down later for his lunchtime nap, he can sleep until between 2.45–3pm.

- Open the curtains, and undo his sleeping bag so that he can wake up naturally. Change his nappy.

- He should be given a breast-feed or a drink of formula milk or water from a beaker and perhaps a snack if he no longer has milk at this time.

- Do not feed baby after 3.15pm as it will put him off his tea.

4.15pm

- Change baby's nappy.

5pm

- Baby should be given most of his solids before being offered a small drink of water or milk from a beaker. It is important that he still has a good milk feed at bedtime, so keep this drink to a minimum.

6.15–6.30pm

- He must start his bath no later than 6.30pm.

- If your baby has several teeth now it is important that enough time is allowed between the milk feed and teeth cleaning. Therefore you can now offer your baby most of his milk feed downstairs before the bath.

6.30pm

- Baby should start his bath no later than 6.30pm.

- He should feed from both breasts or have 210–240ml (7–8oz) of formula milk; this may eventually reduce to 180ml (6oz) when a beaker is introduced at one year. As long as he continues to sleep through to nearer 7am, this is not a problem.

- During bath time or just after, ensure that your baby's teeth are cleaned thoroughly.

- Read a story and offer the remainder of your baby's milk, plus a small drink of water to rinse the milk from his teeth just prior to putting him down to sleep.

7pm

- Settle baby in his sleeping bag, in the dark with the door shut, no later than 7pm.

Changes to be made during the nine- to twelve-month routine

Sleeping

The majority of babies cut back on their daily sleep at this stage. If you notice that your baby is starting to wake in the night or earlier in the morning, it is important that you look at your baby's daytime sleep, so that any reduction in his overall daily sleep needs happens during the day, instead of at night or early morning.

- The first nap to cut back on is the morning one. If he has been having 30 minutes, then try cutting it back to 10–15 minutes. Some babies may also cut back their lunchtime nap to one and a half hours, which can lead to them becoming very tired and irritable late afternoon. If this happens to your baby, try pushing the morning nap later and reduce it to 10–15 minutes. For a short time you may have to bring lunchtime forward slightly if he can't make it through to 12.30pm for his nap.

- If you find that your baby is not going to sleep until nearer 10.30–10.45am, I would restrict the nap to no more than 5–10 minutes to ensure that he settles nearer 12.30pm for his lunch time nap.

- If he does have more than 5-10 minutes at the morning nap he may not be ready to go down for his lunch time nap until 12.45–1pm. This is fine, but if you want him to still be ready for bed at 7pm, I would recommend that you wake him up no later than 2.45pm. If you leave him to sleep until 3pm, he may not be ready to sleep until nearer 7.15–7.30pm.

- If he refuses to have even a very short nap in the morning, you may have to bring the lunch time nap forward slightly.

- Your baby may also start to pull himself up in the cot, but get very upset when he can't get himself back down. If this happens, it would be advisable to put him in the cot standing up to encourage him to practise lying himself down when you put him down for his naps. Until he is able to manoeuvre himself up and down, you will need to go in and help him settle back down. It is important that this is done with the least possible fuss and talking.

- If this is happening, it is also worth taking a look at his daytime sleep total, as repeated waking up and standing up in the night can be a product of too much daytime sleep, which is easily rectified by cutting down, or cutting out, the morning nap (see below).

- Some babies' sleep requirements can change suddenly at 12 months. In order for them to continue sleeping for 12 hours at night, their daytime sleep may need to be cut down to two hours.

Cutting out the morning nap

If you want your baby to continue to sleep well at night and during the lunch time nap, it is really important, if your baby has not already started to do so himself, to begin to reduce the morning nap between nine and 12 months. Gradually push the morning nap on from 9.30am so that your baby is going down nearer to 9.45–10am. Once he is happily going through to this time, gradually reduce the length of nap to 15 minutes. You can then push the lunchtime nap on to nearer 12.45pm and allow a nap of no more than two hours.

- If your baby is showing no signs of being ready to sleep at 9.45–10am, do not be tempted just to drop the morning nap as doing so too early will mean that his lunchtime nap could come too soon, resulting in him going to bed either overtired or too early.

- Keep pushing your baby's nap on until he is managing to get close to 11–11.15am, then allow a nap of no more than 5–10 minutes. Once he is managing to get through to 12.45–1pm for his lunchtime nap with only a 5–10 minute nap at around 11–11.15am, you should be able to cut out the short nap and get him through to 12.15–12.30pm for his lunchtime nap, which can then be increased to two hours.

- If you find that your baby is becoming too tired to eat a proper lunch, you can always bring his lunch forward slightly for a short period until his body clock adjusts to the new nap times. I usually find that once they have had lunch, most babies perk up enough to get through to 12.15–12.30pm.

Feeding

Your baby should be well established on three meals a day, and should also be able to feed himself some of the time. It is very important that your baby learns to chew properly at this stage. Most of his meals should consist of foods that have been chopped, sliced or diced. By the end of his first year he should be able to manage chopped meat. If you have not done so already, nine to twelve months is a good time to introduce raw vegetables and salads. Try to include some finger foods at every meal. Between nine and 12 months it is important to encourage him to feed himself. Using two spoons is a good approach here. Load one spoon with food and put it in his hand whilst gently holding his wrist and encouraging him to get it into his mouth. You can then continue to feed him yourself with the other spoon. Do not discourage these attempts; it is important that he enjoys his meals, even if a certain amount of the food lands on the floor.

- At nine months, a formula-fed baby should be taking all of his water and breakfast milk and 2.30pm feed from a beaker. By the age of one year, he should be drinking all fluids including his bedtime milk from a beaker.

For more information on solid food at this stage see page 279.

15

Introducing Solid Food

Weaning your baby

The latest Department of Health (DoH) guidelines and recommendations from the World Health Organization advise exclusive breast-feeding for the first six months of a baby's life, i.e. no solids or infant formula. The previous DoH advice was to wean between four and six months and not to give solids to any baby before 17 weeks. This is because it takes up to four months for the lining of a baby's gut to develop and for the kidneys to mature enough to cope with the waste products from solid food. If solids are introduced before a baby has the complete set of enzymes required to digest food properly, his digestive system could become damaged.

During the writing of the latest edition of this book, I have spoken to many dieticians and paediatricians as well as to hundreds of mothers via my website. It is clear that there is some controversy surrounding these recommendations. I have found that by speaking to mothers from countries around the world over the last couple of years, that the weaning guidelines in many countries have gone back to advising that babies can be weaned between four to six months. Certainly, there are health professionals who feel that it is not weaning between four and six months which threatens a baby's health, but the kind of food the baby is given. It is also clear that there are many babies who cannot manage on milk alone for the full six months. I urge you to discuss any and all of your concerns with your health visitor or GP and to follow their advice accordingly.

The golden rules are:

- Your baby should not be given food before 17 weeks.

- Weaning should only begin when neuromuscular co-ordination has developed sufficiently, so that the baby can control his head and neck while sitting upright supported in a chair to be fed.

- Your baby should also be able to swallow food easily, by moving it from the front of his mouth to the back.

In this chapter I give a summary of how to introduce solids. For more detailed information, I would recommend *The Contented Little Baby Book of Weaning*, which gives a day-by-day plan for the first two months of weaning to ensure that babies get the correct balance of milk and solids. If you follow the weaning plan in this book and introduce the recommended foods in the order suggested, you can be confident that you are not putting your baby at risk of food allergies.

Babies rely on the introduction of iron-containing foods at six months, as their bodies' iron stores, with which they are born, become depleted at this age. Iron is essential for healthy red blood cells that transport oxygen around the body. Children who do not take in sufficient amounts of iron are at risk of developing iron-deficiency anaemia, which causes tiredness, irritability and an overall lack of energy and enthusiasm. Up to a quarter of 18-month-old children in the UK show signs of iron deficiency anaemia, so if a breast-fed baby is weaned at six months, it is important that iron-containing foods, such as fortified breakfast cereals, broccoli, lentils and baby foods with added iron are introduced swiftly. You will need to progress quickly through the food groups to include meat or pulses for their iron content. Babies on formula will have their iron supplemented in the milk.

I do not know your baby and cannot tell you when he is ready to wean. All babies should be watched closely for signs that they are ready for weaning, which might possibly come sooner than the current DoH recommendations. If your baby is under six months of age and showing all the signs below, it is vital you discuss things with your health visitor or GP and decide with them whether to wean early or not.

I hope the guidelines below will help you identify possible signs of being ready to wean. A baby could be ready if:

- He has been taking a full feed four or five times a day from both breasts or a 240ml (8oz) bottle of formula and has been happily going for four hours between feeds, but now gets irritable and chews his hands long before his next feed is due.

- He has been taking a full feed from both breasts, or a 240ml (8oz) formula feed, and screams for more the minute the feed finishes.

- He usually sleeps well at night and nap times but is starting to wake up earlier and earlier.

- He is chewing his hands excessively, displaying eye-to-hand coordination and trying to put things into his mouth.

If your baby is over four months old, has doubled his birth weight and is consistently displaying most of these signs, he could be ready to begin weaning. If the baby is under six months you should tell your health visitor or GP and decide how to proceed. If you decide to wait until the baby is six months before you introduce solids, it is important that his increased hunger is met by introducing further milk feeds. Babies who have been sleeping through the night with only a small feed at 10.30pm would need to have this feed increased. And, if they go through a further growth spurt before they reach six months, it may be that you need to introduce a further feed in the middle of the night. It is very important to understand that as your baby grows, so will his appetite. If you wish to continue exclusive breast-feeding until six months it is unreasonable to expect the baby to manage on only four milk feeds a day.

Breast-fed babies

With babies who are being breast-fed exclusively it is more difficult to tell how much milk they are receiving. If your baby is over four months and showing most of the above signs, you will need to talk to your health visitor or GP about the choices available to you. If he is under four months and not gaining enough weight each week, it is possible that your milk supply is getting very low in the evening. All that may be needed is extra milk. I suggest you try topping up the baby with 60–90mls (2–3 ounces) of expressed or formula milk after the late feed. If this does not work, or if he is waking up more than once in the night, I would replace the late feed altogether with a full bottle-feed, if you have not already done so. Encourage your partner to do this feed so that you can get to bed early, after expressing whatever milk you have between 9.30–10pm to avoid your supply dropping any further. Mothers in this situation often find that when they express they are only producing 90–120ml (3–4oz), which is much less than their baby may need at this feed. The milk expressed can, if necessary, be given at some other feed during the day, thus avoiding further supplementary bottle-feeding.

This plan usually satisfies a baby's hunger, and improves his weight gain. You should never wean a baby before 17 weeks of age and, if sooner than six months, it should be done only on medical advice.

Foods to be avoided

During the first two years of your baby's life, certain foods are best used sparingly, or avoided altogether, as they may be harmful to your baby's health. The two worst culprits in this regard are sugar and salt.

Sugar

During the first year of weaning, it is best to avoid adding sugar to any of your baby's food, as it may lead to him developing a taste for sweet things. A baby's appetite for savoury foods can be seriously affected if he is allowed lots of food containing sugar or sugar substitutes. But when buying commercial foods these ingredients can be hard to avoid. A survey by the Consumer's Association magazine *Which?* tested 420 baby products and reported that 40 per cent contained sugar or fruit juice or both. When choosing baby cereals or commercial foods, check the labels carefully; sugar may be listed as dextrose, fructose, glucose or sucrose. Watch out, too, for syrup or concentrated fruit juice, which are also sometimes used as sweeteners.

Too much sugar in the diet may not only cause your baby to refuse savoury food, but can lead to serious problems such as tooth decay and obesity. Because sugar converts very quickly into energy, babies and children who have too much may become hyperactive. Products such as baked beans, spaghetti hoops, cornflakes, fish fingers, jam, tomato ketchup, tinned soups and some yoghurts are just a few of the everyday foods that contain hidden sugars, so care should be taken that when your baby reaches toddlerhood he does not eat these foods in excess. It is also important to check the labels of fruit juices and squashes carefully.

Salt

Children under two years of age should not have salt added to their food – they get all the salt they need from natural sources such as vegetables. Adding salt to a young baby's food can be very dangerous, as it may put a strain on his immature kidneys. Research also shows that children with high salt intake may be more prone to heart disease later. When your baby reaches the important stage of joining in with family meals, it is important that you do not add salt to the food during cooking. Remove your baby's portion, then add salt if needed for the rest of the family. As with sugar, many processed foods and commercially prepared meals contain high levels of salt. It is important to check the labels on these foods carefully before giving them to your toddler.

Preparing and cooking food for your baby

Making your own food not only often works out cheaper, but, more importantly, will be of great nutritional benefit for your baby. And it needn't be fiddly or time-consuming if you make up large quantities at a time and store mini meals in the freezer. Keep sterilised feeding equipment, ice cube trays and freezer-proof containers at the ready and follow the general instructions below:

- When preparing food, always ensure that all surfaces are clean and have been wiped down with an anti-bacterial cleaner. Use kitchen roll for cleaning surfaces and drying, as it is more hygienic than kitchen cloths and towels, which may carry bacteria.

- All fresh fruit and vegetables should be carefully peeled, removing the core, pips and any blemishes. They should then be rinsed thoroughly with filtered water.

- If you are advised to wean your baby early, remember that all fruit and vegetables must be cooked until your baby is six months old (apart from banana and avocado). This can be done by either steaming or boiling in filtered water.

- Do not add salt, sugar or honey.

- During the initial stages all food must be cooked until soft enough to purée to a very smooth consistency. A small amount of the cooking water may need to be added so that the mixture is similar to smooth yoghurt.

- If using a food processor, check carefully for lumps by using a spoon and pouring into another bowl. Then transfer to ice cube trays or containers for storage in the freezer.

Sterilised feeding equipment

All feeding equipment should be sterilised for the first six months, and bottles and teats for as long as they are used. Sterilise ice cube trays or freezer containers by boiling them in a large saucepan of water for five minutes. Use a steam steriliser, if you have one, for small items such as spoons or serving bowls, and follow timings recommended in the manufacturer's handbook. Wash cooking utensils as usual in a dishwasher or rinse handwashed items with boiling water from the kettle.

Packing food for the freezer

- Ensure cooked, puréed food is covered as quickly as possible and transfer it to the freezer as soon as it's cool enough.
- Never put warm food into a refrigerator or freezer.
- Check the temperature of your freezer on a freezer thermometer. It should read −18ºC. If you don't have a freezer thermometer, they can be bought from a good hardware shop or the cookware section of a large department store.
- If using an ice cube tray, fill with puréed food, open-freeze until solid, then pop the cubes out of the tray and into a sterilised plastic box. Non-sterilised items such as plastic bags can be used from six months. Seal well and freeze.
- Label items clearly, adding the date.
- Use foods within the Food Standard Agencies guidelines.
- Never refreeze cooked food. Food can only be put back into the freezer if it was originally frozen raw and then defrosted and cooked − a raw frozen chicken breast, defrosted, for example, can be frozen as a cooked casserole.

Defrosting tips

- Defrost frozen (covered) food in the fridge overnight or leave at room temperature if you forget, transferring it to the fridge as soon as it has defrosted. Make sure it is covered at all times and stand it on a plate to catch the drips.

- Never speed up defrosting by putting food into warm or hot water.

- Always use defrosted foods within 24 hours.

Reheating tips

- Food should be heated thoroughly to ensure that any bacteria are killed. If using jars, always transfer to a dish; never serve straight from the jar. Any food left over should be discarded, never reheated and used again.

- When batch-cooking, take out a portion of food for your baby to eat now and freeze the rest. Don't be tempted to reheat the entire mixture and then freeze what is left.

- If your baby has only eaten a tiny portion it can be tempting to reheat and serve leftovers later. Please don't – babies are much more susceptible than adults to food poisoning, so get in the habit of throwing leftovers away immediately.

- Reheat foods only once.

Early weaning

If you have been advised that your baby is ready for weaning before the recommended age of six months, remember that milk is still the most important food for him. It provides him with the right balance of vitamins and minerals. Solids given before six months are classed as first tastes and fillers which should be increased very slowly over several weeks, gradually preparing your baby for three solid meals a day. By offering the milk first you will ensure that his daily milk intake does not decrease too rapidly before he reaches six months.

Studies into weaning by the University of Surrey revealed that babies fed diets with a high fruit content may be more prone to diarrhoea, which leads to slow growth. They advise that baby rice is the best first weaning food as fruit may not be so well tolerated by the under-developed gut of some babies.

Remember that as soon as your baby has teeth and has begun on any type of solid food, he will need his teeth cleaning twice a day.

How to begin

- Introduce solids after the 11am feed. Prepare everything you need for giving the solids in advance: a baby chair, bib, spoon, bowl and a clean, fresh damp cloth.

- Start by offering your baby a teaspoonful of pure organic rice mixed to a very smooth consistency using either expressed milk, formula or cool, filtered, freshly boiled water.

- Make sure the baby rice has cooled enough before feeding it to your baby. Use a shallow plastic spoon for him – never a metal one, which can be too sharp or get too hot.

- Some babies need help in learning how to feed from the spoon. By placing the spoon just far enough into his mouth, and bringing the spoon up and out against the roof of his mouth, his upper gums will take the food off, encouraging him to feed.

- After two of three days of your baby having rice at the 11am feed, you can then offer some pear purée at 11am, and then you can then transfer the rice to the evening. Start off by offering him a small amount of milk around 5pm, followed by the solids, gradually reduce the milk at 5pm, and increase the solids, so that by six months he is having all of his solids at 5pm.

- Once your baby is happily taking 1–2 teaspoonfuls of baby rice mixed with milk or water at 5pm, a small amount of pear purée can be mixed with the baby rice. You should then start to introduce different vegetables at the 11am feed.

- Be guided by your baby as to when to increase the amounts. He will turn his head away and get fussy when he has had enough.

- Mixing the purée with baby rice in the evening will make it more palatable and prevent your baby from getting constipated.

- Small amounts of various organic vegetables and fruit can now be introduced, one by one, after the 11am feed. To prevent your baby from developing a sweet tooth, try to give more vegetables than fruit. At this stage, avoid the stronger-tasting ones such as spinach or broccoli, but rather concentrate on root vegetables such as carrot, sweet potato and swede. These contain natural sugars, will taste sweeter and blander, and may prove more palatable to your baby.

- With babies under six months it is important to introduce new foods in small amounts every 2–3 days. Gradually keep increasing the solids, being guided by your baby. Although all babies are different I have found that the majority of babies are taking around 6 tablespoons of food at lunch and tea between six and seven months. Babies over six months will probably need their meals increased by larger amounts every couple of days, and as long as you stick to the foods recommended for first-stage weaning, you can introduce new foods closer together. Keeping a food diary will help you see how your baby reacts to each new food.

- Always be very positive and smile when offering new foods even if your baby spits it out; it may not mean he dislikes it. Remember this is all very new to him and different foods will get a different reaction. If he positively refuses a food, however, leave it and try again in a week's time.

- Always offer milk first, as this is still the most important food at this stage in nutritional terms. While appetites do vary, in my experience the majority of babies will be taking four to five full feeds of formula or breast milk a day. Provided your baby is happy and thriving, the minimum daily recommended amount of milk required at this age, once solids are established, is 600ml (20oz) a day.

For more comprehensive advice on weaning, including a day-by-day plan for the first two months of weaning, which food to introduce when and how much, as well as recipes you can prepare for your baby, see *The Contented Little Baby Book of Weaning*. There are many more easy-to-prepare recipes for babies and toddlers in *The Gina Ford Baby and Toddler Cook Book* and recipes for all the family, including indispensable meal planners, in *Feeding Made Easy*.

First stage: six to seven months

If your baby started weaning before six months he will probably have tasted baby rice, plus a variety of different vegetables and fruits recommended in the first weaning stage. Follow my guidelines (see page 265) for when to start baby rice and when to introduce fruit and vegetables. Once you have started weaning it is important to keep introducing a variety of the different fruits and vegetables on page 266 in the first-stage weaning foods. Fruit and vegetables should still be steamed or cooked in filtered water until soft, then puréed. Mix to the desired consistency with some of the cooking water, or no-salt chicken stock may be used with some vegetables. You should avoid introducing dairy products, wheat, eggs, nuts and citrus fruit as they are the foods most likely to trigger allergies. Honey should not be introduced before one year. Meat, chicken and fish should not be introduced until the babies are capable of digesting reasonable amounts of other solids. All too often I have seen feeding problems occur because meat, poultry or fish have been introduced too early. Once you have worked through the first foods you can introduce protein. In the meantime, your first sources of iron can be found in lentils, broccoli and iron-fortified breakfast cereals.

When beginning weaning at the age of six months you will need to progress quickly through the first-stage foods so the iron-rich meat and plant protein can be introduced regularly. A rough guideline would be to increase the baby rice at teatime by one teaspoonful of dry rice every couple of days and the savoury at lunchtime by one cube every couple of days. It is also essential to rapidly reduce your baby's milk intake to four feeds a day once solids are established.

Between six and seven months, depending on when you began weaning, your baby should be having 2–3 servings of carbohydrates daily in the form of cereal, wholemeal bread, pasta or potatoes. He should also have three servings of vegetables or fruit each day and one serving of animal or plant protein.

Foods to introduce

Pure organic baby rice, pear, apple, carrot, sweet potato, potato, green beans, courgette and swede are ideal first weaning foods. Once your baby is happily taking these foods, you can introduce parsnip, mango, peach, broccoli, avocado, barley, peas and cauliflower.

Protein in the form of meat, poultry, fish and pulses should be introduced between six and seven months, once your baby is taking around six tablespoons of solids. Check that all the bones are removed and trim off the fat and the skin. Some babies find the flavour of protein cooked on its own too strong.

Try cooking chicken or meat in a casserole with familiar root vegetables, and fish in a milk sauce until your baby becomes accustomed to the different texture and taste. Pulse in a food processor to make it easier for your baby to eat.

Introducing breakfast

A baby is ready to start having breakfast once he shows signs of hunger long before his 11am feed. This usually happens between the ages of six and seven months. Once your baby is eating breakfast, you can gradually start to move the 11am solids until later, eventually settling somewhere between 11.30am and 12 noon. I find that organic oats or millet cereal with a small amount of puréed fruit is a favourite with most babies. By seven months, if your baby is eating a full breakfast of cereal, fruit and perhaps small pieces of toast, you should aim to cut back the amount offered to him from the bottle. Try to give part of the milk as a drink and the remainder with the cereal. Always try to encourage your baby to drink at least 150–180ml milk (5–6oz) before he is given his breakfast solids and then offer any remainder of the milk.

If you are still breast-feeding, ensure that your baby takes the first breast, then give him solids and then offer the second breast. Be very careful not to increase his solids so much that he cuts back too much on his breast-feed.

If your baby reaches seven months and is refusing breakfast, you can always cut back his milk slightly to encourage him to take small amounts of solids.

Regardless of whether you introduced solids before six months or at six months, aim to have a feeding plan similar to the one below before introducing protein. This will ensure that your baby's system is used to digesting reasonable amounts of solids, and can cope with the introduction of protein.

7–7.30am	*Breakfast*
	Breast-feed or 180–240ml (6–8oz) of formula milk.
	2–3 teaspoons of oat cereal mixed with breast milk or formula and 1–2 tablespoons of fruit purée.
11.15–11.30am	*Lunch*
	Breast-feed or give 60–90ml (2–3oz) of formula milk.
	2–3 tablespoons of sweet potato purée and 2–3 tablespoons of root vegetable purée plus 1–2 tablespoons of cauliflower *or* green vegetable purée mixed with some chicken stock.
2–2.30pm	*Mid afternoon*
	Breast-feed or give 150–210ml (5–7oz) formula milk.
	Breast-feed or give 180–240ml (6–8oz) of formula milk.
6pm	*Tea*
	5–6 teaspoons of baby rice mixed with breast milk, formula milk or cool boiled water, mixed with 2 tablespoons of fruit purée.

Introducing protein at lunchtime

If you were advised to wean your baby earlier than normally recommended (see page 259), and if he is eating around six tablespoons of mixed vegetables, you should be able to introduce protein foods as soon as he reaches six months. If you started weaning your baby at six months, it could take between two to three weeks for him to be taking that amount. The best way to introduce the protein is to start off by replacing two of the vegetable cubes with two of the simple chicken, red lentil or fish recipes in *The Contented Little Baby Book of Weaning, The Gina Ford Baby and Toddler Cook Book* and *Feeding Made Easy*. Introduce new protein foods slowly at this stage – one every three days is about right. If your baby has no reaction, then keep replacing one or two cubes of vegetables every day until the six cubes of vegetables are replaced with a complete protein recipe. Once your baby is taking a full protein meal at lunchtime, it is important to introduce him to a beaker at lunchtime. Once protein is introduced at lunchtime and your baby is eating around six tablespoons of solids, his milk intake after the solids should have reduced to just two or three ounces (60–90ml). At this stage it is important to start to offer a small drink of water midway through his meal and at the end of his meal, eventually dropping the milk feed altogether. However, if you find your baby starts to wake up slightly earlier from his lunchtime nap, you can offer a small milk feed just prior to the nap for a further few weeks.

Once the lunchtime milk is dropped, he may need to increase the 2.30pm feed. However, if you notice that he is cutting back too much on his teatime solids or bedtime feed, continue to keep this feed smaller. Between six and seven months, once protein meals are established at lunchtime, milk at 5 pm and the baby rice and fruit should gradually be replaced with a savoury meal, with only a small drink of water from a beaker. You would then give your baby a full milk feed around 6.30pm.

Introducing a beaker

Once protein is well established, your baby's milk feed should be replaced at lunchtime by a drink of cool boiled water from a beaker. Most babies are capable of sipping and swallowing at this age, and this should be encouraged by being consistent and always offering the lunchtime drink from a beaker. Do not worry if your baby only drinks a small amount at this meal. You will probably find that he makes up for it at his 2.30pm feed or takes an increase of cool boiled water later in the day. If you find that your baby's sleeping becomes unsettled at lunchtime when you drop the milk feed, you may for a short time have to go back to offering him a small top-up of milk prior to the lunchtime nap, but it is important that you keep persevering with offering him fluids from his beaker at lunchtime.

Tea/dinner

If you always make sure that your baby has a well-balanced breakfast and lunch you can be relaxed about this meal. Once breakfast and lunch are established, you can sit the baby down at 5pm and offer him a small tea. Some babies can get very fractious around this time of the day, so offer foods that are quick and easy to prepare – thick vegetable soups and vegetable bakes that have been prepared and frozen in advance are always a good standby. Pasta, or a baked potato, served with vegetables and a sauce is also nutritious and easy. A very hungry baby can also be offered a milk pudding or yoghurt.

Daily requirements

By six months a baby who started weaning early will probably be established on two solid meals a day, and between six and seven months, it is important that you work towards establishing your baby on three proper meals a day. These should include three servings of carbohydrates, such as cereals, bread and pasta, plus at least three servings of vegetables and fruit, and one serving of puréed meat or fish or two servings of pulses. By six months a baby has used up most of the iron stores he was born with. As their iron requirements between six and twelve months are particularly high, it is important that their diet provides the right amount of this mineral. To help iron absorption in cereals and meat, always serve with fruit or vegetables rich in vitamin C. Getting the balance of solids right is vital, so that he continues to get the right amount of milk. Although he will have cut down on the 11am breast- or bottle-feed of milk as his intake of solids increases, he still needs a minimum of 500–600ml (18–20oz) of breast or formula milk a day, inclusive of milk used for mixing food. Babies who started weaning at six months could still be having

4–5 milk feeds a day, which you need to reduce rapidly if solids are not to be refused. Some babies who are still drinking large amounts of milk at six months may be resistant to the introduction of solids. If you find that your baby is fussy about taking solids you should only offer him a very small amount of milk at the 11am feed to encourage interest in the solid food. You should aim to have your baby on two meals a day within a couple of weeks of beginning solids. By the time he reaches seven months, regardless of when he began weaning, all babies should be well-established on two meals a day, progressing to three meals consisting of a wide variety of foods from the different food groups. At the end of six months a typical day's menu may look something like this:

7–7.30am *Breakfast*

Breast-feed or 150–240ml (5–8oz) of formula milk, 60–90ml (2–3oz) of which to be mixed with cereal. 4–6 teaspoons of dry oat cereal mixed with milk and fruit *or* toast with fruit spread.

11.30am *Lunch*

6 tablespoons chicken casserole *or* vegetable and lentil shepherd's pie *or* steamed fish with creamed vegetables. Small drink of water from a beaker.

2.30pm *Mid-afternoon*

Breast-feed or 120–210ml (4–7oz) of formula milk. If your baby is still having a small drink of milk prior to the lunch time nap, offer less at this feed, so as not to reduce appetite for 5pm solids.

5pm *Tea*

6 tablespoons baked potato with creamed vegetables *or* pasta with red pepper sauce. Cheese, rice cakes or yoghurt. Small drink of water from a beaker.

6.30pm Breast-feed or 210–240ml (7–8oz) of formula milk.

Once a baby is established on three good solid meals a day, plus three or four full milk feeds, he should manage to go nearer to 12 hours without a feed. If your baby is not cutting down on his late feed once solids are introduced, it may be that he is not getting the right quantities of solids for his age or weight, or too small a feed at 6.30pm. Keep a diary of all food and milk consumed over a period of four days to help pinpoint why he is not cutting that last feed.

By the end of six months your baby will probably be ready to sit in a high chair for his meals. Always ensure that he is properly strapped in and never left unattended.

Second stage: seven to nine months

During the second stage of weaning, the amount of milk your baby drinks will gradually reduce as his intake of solids increases. It is, however, important that he still receives a minimum of 500–600ml (18–20oz) a day of breast or formula milk. This is usually divided between three milk feeds and milk used in food and cooking. At this stage of weaning you should be aiming at establishing three good solid meals a day, so that by the time your baby reaches nine months of age he is getting most of his nourishment from solids. During this time it is important to keep introducing a wide variety of foods from the different food groups (carbohydrate, protein, dairy, fruit and vegetables) so that your baby's nutritional needs are met. Most babies are ready to accept stronger-tasting foods at this age. They also take pleasure from different textures, colours and presentation. Foods should be mashed or 'pulsed' and kept separate to avoid mixing everything up. Fruit need not be cooked; it can be grated or mashed. It is also around this age that your baby will begin to put food in his mouth. Raw soft fruit, lightly cooked vegetables and toast can be used as finger foods. They will be sucked and squeezed more than eaten at this stage, but allowing your baby the opportunity to feed himself encourages good feeding habits later on. Once your baby is having finger foods, always wash his hands before a meal and *never* leave him alone while he is eating.

During the second stage of weaning, when your baby increases the types of foods that he eats, you can start to plan meals that are suitable for all the family. When giving your baby casseroles, you will still have to purée or pulse the meat: simply remove a portion of the meat, along with a little of the liquid, and purée or pulse to a texture that your baby will accept. Then serve with the appropriate amount of vegetables in the casserole. At this stage you may still have to chop or slice the vegetables smaller, but it is important that you start to move away from serving whole meals pulsed or puréed.

See *The Contented Little Baby Book of Weaning* for examples of the types of meals that you can plan for your baby during the second stage of weaning.

Between eight and nine months your baby may show signs of wanting to use his spoon. To encourage this, use two spoons when you feed him. Load one for him to try and get the food into his mouth. You use the other for actually getting the food in! You can help your baby's co-ordination by holding his wrist gently and guiding the spoon into his mouth. Finger foods should also be offered at every meal at this stage.

Foods to introduce

Dairy products, pasta and wheat can be introduced at this stage. Full-fat cow's milk can be used in cooking, but should not be given as a drink until one year. Small amounts of unsalted butter can also be used in cooking. Egg yolks can be introduced, but must be hard-boiled. Cheese should be full-fat, pasteurised and grated, and preferably organic. Olive oil can be used when cooking casseroles.

Canned fish such as tuna may also be included, but choose fish in vegetable or olive oil, as fish canned in brine has a higher salt content. A greater variety of vegetables can also be introduced, such as peppers, Brussels sprouts, pumpkin, cabbage, tomatoes and spinach. All these foods should be introduced gradually and careful notes made of any reactions. Once your baby is used to taking food from a spoon, vegetables can be mashed rather than puréed. Once he is happy taking mashed food you can start to introduce small amounts of finger food. Vegetables should be cooked until soft then offered in cube-sized pieces or steamed and then mixed to the right consistency. Once your baby is managing softly cooked pieces of vegetables and soft pieces of raw fruit, you can try him with toast or rice cakes. By nine months, if your baby has several teeth he should be able to manage some chopped raw vegetables.

Breakfast

Low-sugar cereals can now be introduced; choose those fortified with iron and B vitamins. Try to alternate the cereals between oat-based and wheat-based, even if your baby shows a preference for one over the other. You may want to delay introducing these if you have a family history of allergies – check with your health visitor, GP or a dietician. Try adding a little mashed or grated fruit if your baby refuses them. You can encourage your baby with finger foods by offering him a little buttered toast at this stage. Once your baby is finger-feeding, you can offer a selection of fruits and yoghurts along with lightly buttered toast.

Most babies are still keen for their milk first thing in the morning, so allow him two-thirds of his milk first. Once he is nearer nine months of age he will most likely show signs of not being hungry for milk and this is the time to try offering breakfast milk from a beaker.

Lunch

If your baby is eating a proper breakfast you will be able to push lunch to somewhere between 11.45am and 12 noon. However, should he be eating only a small amount of breakfast, lunch will need to come slightly earlier. Likewise, babies who are having only a very short nap in the morning may also need to have lunch earlier. It's important to remember that overtired, hungry babies will not feed as well, so take your timing of lunch from your baby.

During this stage of weaning you will have established protein at lunchtime. Whenever possible, try to buy organic meat as this is free from additives and growth stimulators. Pork, bacon and processed hams should not be introduced until 18 months as they have a high salt content. You should still continue to cook without additional salt or sugar (see page 260 for foods to avoid), although a small amount of herbs and spices can be introduced at around nine months of age.

If you are introducing your baby to a vegetarian diet, it is important to seek expert advice on getting the right balance of amino acids. Vegetables are incomplete sources of amino acids when cooked separately and need to be combined correctly to provide your baby with a complete source of protein. Once protein is well-established, your baby's milk feed should be replaced at lunchtime by a drink of cool, boiled water from a beaker. You might find that he only drinks a small amount from the beaker and looks for an increase of milk on the 2.30pm feed or an increase of cool, boiled water later in the day. If your baby is still hungry after his main meal, offer a piece of cheese, a breadstick, rice cake or yoghurt.

Tea

Once your baby is finger-feeding, tea can include a selection of mini-sandwiches. Baked potatoes or pasta served with vegetables and sauces are also suitable, although he will need help eating these. Some babies get very tired and fussy by teatime. If your baby does not eat much, try offering some rice pudding, cereal or carrot or banana cake. A small drink of water from a beaker can be offered after the tea. Do not allow too large a drink at this time as it will put him off his last milk feed. His bedtime milk feed is still important at this stage. If he starts cutting back too much on this feed, check you are not overfeeding him on solids or giving him too much to drink.

Daily requirements

At this second stage of weaning it is important that you work towards establishing your baby on three proper meals a day. They should include three servings of carbohydrates, such as cereals, bread and pasta, plus at least three servings of vegetables and fruit, and one serving of puréed meat, fish or pulses. By six months a baby has used up all the store of iron he was born with. As their requirements between six and twelve months are particularly high, it is important that their diet provides the right amount of iron.

Your baby still needs 500–600ml (18–20oz) of breast or formula milk a day, inclusive of milk used for mixing food. If your baby starts to reject his milk, try reducing the amount of solids you give him at teatime. By the end of nine months try to encourage your baby to drink all of his breakfast milk from a beaker. Apart from his bedtime milk, all other milk feeds and drinks should ideally be from a beaker.

A very hungry baby who is taking three full milk feeds a day, plus three solid meals, may need a small drink and a piece of fruit mid-morning.

A typical day's menu for an eight- to nine-month-old baby would look like this:

7–7.30am	*Breakfast* Breast-feed or 150–180ml (5–6oz) of formula milk in a beaker. Mixed mashed fruit and yoghurt or wheat/oat cereal with milk and mashed fruit.
11.45am	*Lunch* Chicken, broccoli and pasta in a cream sauce *or* Fish cakes with cabbage and carrots. Fruit and yoghurt. Drink of water from a beaker.
2.30pm	*Mid-afternoon* Breast-feed or 120–180ml (4–6oz) of formula milk in a beaker.
5pm	*Tea* Baked potato with grated cheese and apple *or* Vegetable lasagne. Drink of water from a beaker.
6.30pm	Breast-feed or 210–240ml (7–8oz) of formula milk.

Third stage: nine to twelve months

Between nine and twelve months your baby should be eating and enjoying all types of food, with the exception of food with a high fat, salt or sugar content. Peanuts and honey should also still be avoided. It is very important that your baby learns to chew properly at this stage. Food should be chopped or diced, although meat may still need to be pulsed. By the end of his first year, he should be able to manage chopped meat. This is also a good time to introduce raw vegetables and salads. Try to include some finger foods at every meal, and if he shows an interest in holding his own spoon, do not discourage these attempts. When he repeatedly puts it in his mouth, load up another spoon and let him try to get it into his mouth, quickly popping in any food that falls out with your spoon. With a little help and guidance, from 12 months most babies are capable of feeding themselves with part of their meal. It is important to encourage self-feeding even if a certain amount of it lands on the floor.

Breakfast

Aim to get your baby to have 200ml (7oz) of milk at this meal, divided between a drink and his breakfast cereal. Scrambled egg can be offered once or twice a week as a change. Ensure that you still offer milk at the start of the meal. Once he has taken 150–180ml (5–6oz) of his milk, offer him some cereal. Then offer him the remainder of his milk again. It is important that he has at least 180–240ml (6–8oz) of milk divided between the beaker and the breakfast cereal. If you are still breast-feeding, offer him the first breast then the solids, then offer him the breast again. Between nine and 12 months, a baby needs a minimum of 500ml (18oz) a day (inclusive of milk used in cooking or in cereal) divided between two or three milk feeds. This total also includes yoghurt and cheese – as a guide, a 125g (4oz) pot of yoghurt or a 30g (1oz) piece of cheese is the equivalent of approximately 210ml (7oz) of milk.

Lunch

Lunch should consist of a wide selection of lightly steamed chopped vegetables, a serving of carbohydrate in the form of potato, pasta or rice, and a serving of protein. Babies of this age are very active and can become quite tired and irritable by 5pm. By ensuring a well-balanced lunch, you will not need to worry if tea is more relaxed. By the end of the first year your baby's lunch can be integrated with the family lunch. Prepare the meal without salt, sugar or spices, reserve a portion for your baby and then add the desired flavourings for the rest of the family. Try to ensure that his meals are attractively presented, with a variety of different-coloured vegetables and fruit. Do not overload his plate; serve up a small amount and, when he finishes that, replenish his plate. This also helps to avoid the game of throwing food on the floor, which often occurs at this stage. If your baby does start to play up with his main course, refusing to eat and throwing food around, quietly and firmly say 'stop' and remove the plate. Do *not* offer him a biscuit or yoghurt half an hour later, as a pattern will soon emerge where he will refuse lunch knowing he will get something sweet if he plays up enough. A piece of fruit can be offered mid-afternoon to see him through to tea, at which time he will probably eat very well.

A drink of well-diluted, pure, unsweetened orange juice in a beaker will help the absorption of iron at this meal, but make sure your baby has most of his meal before you allow him to finish the drink.

The 2.30pm feed

By nine to 12 months, bottle-fed babies should be given most of their milk from a beaker, which should automatically result in a decrease in the amount they drink. If your baby starts to cut back on his last milk feed, reduce the 2.30pm feed. Many babies cut out the 2.30pm feed by one year. At 12 months, as long as your baby is getting a minimum of 350ml (12oz) of milk a day, inclusive of milk used in cereal and cooking, he will be getting enough. If he is getting 540ml (18oz) of milk a day (inclusive of milk used in cooking, on cereal, plus a full balanced diet of solids, you could cut this feed altogether. Once your baby has dropped this feed, it can be replaced by a small snack (for example a rice cake/unsweetened biscuit or small piece of fruit) and a drink of water from a beaker.

Tea

Many babies cut out their 2.30pm milk during this stage. If you are worried that your baby's daily milk intake is too low, try giving him things like pasta and vegetables with a milk sauce, baked potatoes with grated cheese, cheesy vegetable bake or mini quiches at teatime. Teatime is usually the meal when I would give small helpings of milk pudding or yoghurt, which are also alternatives if milk is being rejected. Try regularly to include some finger foods at teatime.

The bedtime bottle should be discouraged after one year, so during this stage get your baby gradually used to less milk at bedtime. This can be done by offering him a small drink of milk with his teatime meal, then a drink of 150–180ml (5–6oz) of milk from a beaker at bedtime.

The 6–7pm feed

By 10–12 months, bottle-fed babies should be taking all of their milk from a beaker. Babies who continue to feed from a bottle after one year are more prone to feeding problems, as they continue to take large amounts of milk, which takes the edge off their appetite for solids.

Start encouraging your baby to take some of his milk from a beaker at nine months, so that by one year he is happy to give up his bottles.

Daily requirements

By one year it is important that large volumes of milk are discouraged; no more than 600ml (20oz), inclusive of milk used in food, should be allowed. More than this can adversely affect his appetite for solid food. After one year your baby needs a minimum of 350ml (12oz) a day. This is usually divided between two or three drinks and is inclusive of milk used in cooking or on cereals. Full-fat, pasteurised cow's milk can be given to drink after one year. If your baby refuses cow's milk, try gradually diluting his formula with it until he is happy to take full cow's milk. If possible try to give your baby organic cow's milk as it comes from cows fed exclusively on grass and therefore has more Omega 3 essential fatty acids than non-organic milk. Omega 3 fatty acids are essential for maintaining a healthy heart, supple and flexible joints, healthy growth and strong bones and teeth so it is important to make sure your baby is getting enough of them through his food. All bottles or beakers used for formula milk should still be sterilised until your baby is 12 months old.

Aim to give your baby three well-balanced meals a day and avoid snacks of biscuits, cakes and crisps. Every day aim for him to have three to four servings of carbohydrate, three to four servings of vegetables and fruit, and one portion of animal protein or two of vegetable protein.

By one year your baby's menu should look something like this:

7–7.30am   *Breakfast*
Breast-feed or a drink of formula milk in a beaker.
Wholewheat or oat cereal with milk and fruit *or* Baby muesli with milk and fruit *or* Scrambled egg on toast *or* Yoghurt and chopped fruit.

12 noon   *Lunch*
Cold, creamed chicken with apple and celery salad *or* Beef meatballs in tomato sauce with cabbage and mashed potatoes *or* Tuna burgers and mixed vegetables *or* Irish stew with parsley dumplings.
Drink of water from a beaker.
Yoghurt cheese, breadsticks and rice cakes.

2.30pm   *Mid-afternoon*
Drink of milk, water or well-diluted juice from a beaker.

5pm   *Tea*
            Thick soup and savoury sandwiches *or* vegetarian pizza
            with green salad *or* chickpea and spinach croquettes
            with a homemade tomato sauce *or* lentil and vegetable
            lasagne.
            Small drink of milk, water from a beaker.
6.30pm   Breast-feed or 180ml (6oz) of formula or cow's milk from
            a beaker.

Your questions answered

Q How will I know when my baby is ready to be weaned?

- If your baby has been sleeping through and starts to wake up
  in the night or very early in the morning, and will not settle
  back to sleep unless fed.

- A bottle-fed baby would be taking in excess of 960–1140ml
  (32–38oz) a day, draining a 240ml (8oz) bottle each feed and
  looking for another feed long before it is due.

- A breast-fed baby would start to look for a feed every 2–3
  hours.

- Both breast- and bottle-fed babies would start to chew on
  their hands a lot and be very irritable in between feeds.

- If unsure, always talk to your health visitor or paediatrician,
  especially if your baby is less than six months old.

Q At what milk feed should I introduce solids?

- Milk is still the most important source of food so it's best to
  ensure that your baby has had two full milk feeds in the day
  before offering solids. I usually recommend starting solids

at the 11am feed as this feed will gradually be pushed to 12 noon, becoming a proper lunch once solids become established.

- By giving solids after this feed you can be sure that your baby will have at least half of his daily milk intake before noon.

- If a very hungry baby has no adverse reaction to the baby rice within three days, I would then transfer the rice to after the 5pm milk feed.

Q Which is the best food to introduce?

- I find pure organic baby rice is the food that satisfies most babies' hunger the best. If this is tolerated I would then introduce some organic puréed pear.

- Once these two foods are established, it is best to concentrate on introducing a variety of first-stage vegetables.

- In a survey carried out by the University of Surrey it was found that babies weaned on fruit were less likely to thrive than babies weaned on baby rice. They advise that all babies should start weaning on baby rice.

Q How will I know how much solid food to give my baby?

- For the first six months, milk is still the most important part of your baby's diet. It will provide him with the right balance of vitamins and minerals, so once solids are introduced he will need a minimum of 600ml (20oz) a day. During the first weeks of weaning, if you always offer the milk feed first, then the solids, you can be sure he will take exactly the amount of solids he needs. This avoids him replacing his milk too quickly with solids.

- Once you have established rice and some purées you can start at the 11am feed to give half the milk feed first, then some solids followed by more milk. This will encourage your baby to cut back slightly on his milk feed and increase his solids, preparing him for a feeding pattern of three meals a day at seven months.

- For breast-fed babies, a feed from one breast can be classed as half a milk feed.

Q At what age do I start to cut out milk feeds and which ones do I cut first?

- Assuming your baby was on five milk feeds when he started to wean, once he increases his solids, he should automatically cut back on his late feed, then cut it out altogether. If you wean at six months, you will probably need to keep the late feed. Once solids are established it should be easy to cut out.

- Assuming your baby was sleeping through the night from his late feed on five milk feeds when he started to wean, the first milk feed that should be dropped would be the late feed.

- As your baby increases his day time solids this late feed should automatically reduce the amount he drinks at the late feed. Once he is fully weaned taking around six to eight tablespoons of solids three times a day, he should not need a late feed, provided he is taking a full milk feed at bedtime.

- If he is not showing signs of wanting to drop the late feed, you can gradually reduce the amount he has every few nights. If he continues to sleep through on just a very small feed, it can then be dropped altogether.

- If your baby is breast fed and still waking up around 5am, despite being fed at the late feed, it is probably worth trying to drop the late feed and see if he still sleeps nearer to 5am. At least this way it means he is only having one feed in the 12-hour night.

- The next feed to be dropped would be the 11–11.30am milk feed. As your baby increases his solids this feed should automatically reduce and once he is having six to eight tablespoons of a protein-based meal at lunch then the milk feed should be replaced with a drink of water from a beaker. However, if you find that your baby starts to wake up earlier from his lunch time nap I would advise that you continue to offer him a small milk feed just prior to his lunch time nap.

- The 2.30pm feed often increases for a few months then, somewhere between nine and 12 months, he may lose interest in this feed, at which time it can be dropped.

- Once the 11–11.30am milk feed is dropped the 2.30pm milk feed often increases. However, keep a close eye that you do not increase it so much that it reduced his appetite for tea time solids and his bedtime milk feed.

- If a baby continues to have a small milk feed just prior to his lunch time nap, he will probably only take a small amount at the 2.30pm feed. This is fine, it is important that you do not feed him later than 2.30–3pm as this could affect his appetite for his tea time solids and his bedtime milk feed.

- Between nine and 12 months many babies lose interest in their 2.30pm milk feed; if this is the case you can offer your baby a drink of water and a snack mid-afternoon. If you find that he is still taking a big feed at 2.30pm and reducing the amount he drinks at bedtime, it would be wise to reduce and cut out the 2.30pm milk feed.

Q At what age would you introduce a drinking beaker and at which feeds?

- Between the age of six and seven months is the best time.

- When you have replaced the lunchtime milk feed with water, try giving it from a beaker or a bottle with a hard spout.

- Try halfway through the meal and after every few spoonfuls of food.

- It is important to persevere. Experiment with different types of beaker until you find one with which your baby is happy.

- Once he is taking a few ounces from a beaker, gradually introduce it at other feeds.

Q When can I introduce cow's milk?

- It is recommended that a small amount of cow's milk can be used in cooking from six months.

- Cow's milk should not be given as a drink until your baby is at least one year old.

- It should always be full-fat, pasteurised milk, preferably organic.

- If your baby refuses cow's milk, try reducing the formula by 30ml (1oz) and replacing it with cow's milk. Once he is happy taking that, gradually increase the cow's milk until he is happy with all cow's milk.

Q At what age can I stop puréeing my baby's food?

- Once your baby has taken well to puréed food (hopefully by the end of the sixth month), you can start to mash or pulse the vegetables and fruit really well, so that there are no lumps, but it is not as smooth as the puréed food.

- Between six and nine months I gradually mash and pulse the food less and less until the babies will take food with more texture. It is also important to serve food chopped, sliced and diced. Also include lots of finger foods at this stage.

- Some babies may need their chicken and meat pulsed until they are between ten and twelve months old.

Q When will he be able to spoon-feed himself?

- Once your baby starts to grab at the spoon, give him one to hold.
- When he repeatedly puts it in his mouth, load up another spoon and let him try to get it into his mouth, quickly popping in any food that falls out with your spoon.
- With a little help and guidance, most babies from 12 months are capable of feeding themselves with part of their meal.
- Always supervise your baby during mealtimes. Never, ever leave him alone.

Q When can I stop sterilising?

- Bottles should be sterilised until your baby is one year old.
- Dishes and spoons can stop being sterilised when your baby is six months old. Then put them in the dishwasher, or wash thoroughly in hot soapy water, rinse and leave to air-dry.
- After six months, the pots, cooking utensils and ice cube trays used for preparing weaning food can either be put in the dishwasher or washed in hot soapy water, rinsed and then have boiled water poured over them before being left to air-dry.

Q Which foods are most likely to cause allergies and what are the main symptoms?

- The most common foods that cause allergies are dairy products, wheat, fish, eggs and citrus fruits.

- Symptoms include rashes, wheezing, coughing, runny nose, sore bottom, diarrhoea, irritability and swelling of the eyes.

- Keeping a detailed record when you are weaning can be a big help when you are trying to establish the cause of any of the above symptoms.

- The above symptoms can also be caused by the house mite, animal fur, wool and certain soaps and household cleaning agents.

- If in doubt, always check with your doctor to rule out any other possible causes or illness for the above symptoms.

16

Problem-Solving in the First Year

The advice in this book is based on the hundreds of babies I have personally cared for. However, each baby is an individual and it is natural that problems may occur. Drawing on the feedback from thousands of consultations, I have focused on the most common problems encountered by parents during the first year, and this chapter should cover the majority of your concerns. Remember to consult your doctor or health visitor with any worries – even if they seem small and you fear looking like a neurotic parent. It's better that you are not beset with worries and can enjoy your baby and this precious first year together. You can use the list of headings on the contents page (pages v–viii) to find the problems that concern you. I have divided the information into three sections – general, feeding and sleeping problems – but many of them overlap. Sleeping and feeding are interdependent so you may find it more helpful to read this entire chapter.

General problems

Burping

It is important to follow your baby's lead regarding when to stop and wind him during feeding. If you constantly interrupt his feed to try and get his wind up, he will be more likely to get so upset and frustrated that the crying will cause more wind than the feed itself. Time and time again I watch babies being patted endlessly on the back, the mother refusing to continue with the feed as she is convinced the baby has wind. The reality is that very few babies need to be burped more than once during a feed and once at the end.

A breast-feeding baby will pull himself off the breast when he is ready to burp. If he has not done so by the end of the first breast, you can try burping him before putting him on the second breast. Bottle-fed babies will normally drink half to three-quarters of their feed and pull themselves off to be burped. Regardless of whether you are breast-feeding or bottle-feeding, if you adopt the correct holding position as illustrated on pages 62 and 79, your baby should bring his wind up quickly and easily both during and at the end of the feed. If your baby does not bring up the wind within a few minutes it is best to leave it and try later. More often than not he will bring it up after he has been laid flat for his nappy change.

Occasionally, a baby passing excessive wind from his bottom can suffer considerable discomfort and become very distressed. A breast-feeding mother should keep a close eye on her diet to see if a particular food or drink is causing the wind. Citrus fruits or drinks taken in excess can sometimes cause severe wind in some babies. The other culprits are chocolate and excessive dairy intake. Special care should be taken to make sure that the baby is reaching the hind milk. Too much fore milk can cause explosive bowel movements and excessive passing of wind. With a bottle-fed baby who is already feeding from special anti-colic bottles, the cause of excessive wind is usually overfeeding. If your baby is regularly drinking 90–180ml (3–6oz) a day more than the amount advised on the tin, and constantly putting on in excess of 240g (8oz) of weight each week, cut back on a couple of his feeds (either the 2.30pm or 5pm) for a few days to see if there is any improvement. A 'sucky' baby could be offered a dummy after the smaller feeds to satisfy his sucking needs. Sometimes a teat with a hole either too small or too large for your baby's needs can cause excessive wind. Experiment with the different sizes of teats; sometimes using a smaller hole at a couple of the feeds can help a baby who is drinking some of his feeds too quickly.

Colic

Colic is a common problem for babies under three months. The term colic refers to a baby who screams constantly often for hours at a time, usually in the evening, but where no medical explanation can be given. It can make life miserable for the baby and the parents, and to date there is no cure for it. There are over-the-counter medications, but most parents with a baby suffering from severe colic say that they are of little help. Although a baby can suffer from colic at any time of the day, the most common time seems to be between 6pm and midnight. Parents resort to endless feeding, rocking, patting, driving the baby round the block, most of which seem to bring little or no relief. Colic usually disappears by four months of age, but by that time the baby has often learned all the wrong sleep associations, so the parents are no further forward.

Parents who contact me for help with their 'colicky' baby describe how the baby screams, often for hours at a time, thrashes madly and keeps bringing his legs up in pain. These babies seem to have one thing in common: they are all being fed on demand. Feeding this way all too often leads to the baby having a feed before the first one has been digested, one of the factors that I believe may cause colic. (See also the advice on feeding bottles on page 21.) Not one of the babies I have cared for has ever suffered from colic and I am convinced that it is because I structured their feeding and sleeping from day one.

When I'd go in to help an older baby who was suffering from colic it seemed to disappear within 24 hours of them being put on to the routine.

With breast-fed babies I would often find that excessive crying in the evening was due to genuine hunger, as the mother's milk supply is often lower in the evening. By getting her to express a little milk earlier in the day and topping up with the expressed milk after the bath, more often than not the babies would settle quickly. With bottle-fed babies the excessive crying was rarely due to hunger, and overtiredness was usually the cause. With both breast-fed and bottle-fed babies, I would recommend an earlier bedtime of around 6.15–6.30pm for a few nights to see if overtiredness was the cause. Once you are confident that neither hunger nor tiredness is the reason your baby is still not settling well in the evening, I would recommend that for several nights you try the Assisting to sleep method on page 337. This is a gentle way of resetting your baby's body clock so that he sleeps at the right times and I have found it hugely successful with babies who are really unsettled in the evening. With breast-fed babies, to rule out possible hunger as a cause of evening crying, I would recommend that you offer a top-up of expressed milk after the bath in conjunction with doing the assisted to sleep method.

Crying

I have read in many leading baby books that most young babies cry on average for a total of two hours in a day. This is also the information given by the Thomas Coram Research Unit at London University. They also claim that at six weeks crying reaches a peak, with 25 per cent of babies crying and fussing for at least four hours a day. Dr St James-Roberts also claims that 40 per cent of the crying occurs between 6pm and midnight. Dutch researchers Van de Rijt and Plooij, authors of *Why They*

Cry: Understanding Child Development in the First Year, have spent over 20 years studying baby development and they claim that babies become troublesome and demanding when they are going through one of the seven major neurological changes that occur during the first year.

With very young babies I have noticed that they do go through a more unsettled stage around three weeks and six weeks, which tends to coincide with growth spurts. However, I would be absolutely horrified if any of my babies cried for even one hour a day, let alone 2–4 hours! The one thing that parents comment upon time and time again is how happy their baby is on the routine. Of course, my babies do cry; some when they have their nappy changed, others when having their faces washed, and a few try to fight sleep when put in their cots. With the ones that fight sleep, because I know that they are well fed, burped and ready to sleep, I am very strict. I let them fuss and yell for 10–12 minutes until they have settled themselves. This is the only real crying I experience, and even then it is with the minority of my babies and lasts for no longer than a week or two. Understandably, all parents hate to hear their baby cry; many are worried that to put their baby down in a cot to sleep and leave him to cry like this could be psychologically damaging. I would like to reassure you that, provided your baby has been well fed, and that you have followed the routines regarding awake periods and wind-down time, your baby will not suffer psychological damage. In the long term you will have a happy, contented baby who has learned to settle himself to sleep. Many parents who have followed the demand method with the first baby, and my routines with their second baby, would confirm whole-heartedly that my methods are by far the best and, in the long term, the easiest.

Marc Weissbluth MD, Director of the Sleep Disorders Center at the Children's Memorial Hospital, Chicago, says in his book, *Healthy Sleep Habits, Happy Child*, that parents should remember they are *allowing* their baby to cry, not *making* him cry. He also says that it will be much harder for an older baby to learn how to settle himself. Therefore, do not feel guilty or cruel if you have to allow a short spell of crying when your baby is going off to sleep. He will very quickly learn to settle himself, as long as you have made sure he is well fed, and has been awake enough, but not so long that he becomes overtired.

Listed below are the main reasons a healthy baby would cry. Use it as checklist to eliminate the possible cause for your baby crying. At the top of the list is hunger. A tiny baby who is hungry should always be fed, regardless of the routines.

Hunger

When your baby is very tiny and fretful and unsettled, it is of course wise to assume that when he cries the problem is hunger and to offer him a feed, even if it is before the time recommended in the routine for his age. One of the main reasons that I find very young breast-fed babies are unsettled in the evening is often hunger. If your baby feeds well, stays awake for a short spell after feeds, then sleeps well until the next feed, but is unsettled in the evening – it is very possible the cause is hunger. Even if your baby is putting on a good amount of weight each week, you should not rule out hunger. Many mothers I know can produce a lot of milk early on in the day, but come the evening, when tiredness has crept in, the milk supply can decrease dramatically. I would strongly recommend that, for a few nights, you try topping him up with a small amount of expressed milk after his bath. If he settles well then you will know that your milk supply is low at that time of the evening. Please check page 313 for suggestions on how to deal with this problem.

However, if you find that your baby is unsettled in the evening, or indeed any other time of the day, despite being well fed, it is important that you try to eliminate other reasons for him being fretful. All too often I hear people saying that it is normal for babies to cry a lot in the early days as 'that is what babies do'. During my many years of caring for young babies, I did have some who indeed were very fretful in the early days, no matter what I did to try and help calm them. But I have to stress that out of the hundreds of babies I cared for, there could only have been a handful. If I found that I had a very unsettled baby I would go through every possibility before accepting that there was nothing I could do to help improve things. Babies do have many needs other than feeding, sleeping and being held.

Tiredness

Babies under six weeks tend to get tired after one hour of being awake. Although they may not be quite ready to sleep, they need to be kept quiet and calm. Not all babies show obvious signs of tiredness, so, in the early days, after they have been awake for one hour, I would still advise you to take them somewhere quiet so they can wind down gradually. Try not to allow visitors to overstimulate them during this wind-down period.

Overtiredness

Very young babies should not be allowed to stay awake for more than two hours at a time, as they can become very overtired and difficult to settle. If your baby is not settling well in the evening it is worth considering that he could be overtired and try settling him in his bed earlier around 6.15–6.30pm.

Overtiredness is often a result of overstimulation. An overtired baby reaches a stage where he is unable to drift off to sleep naturally, and the more tired he becomes, the more he fights sleep. A baby under three months who is allowed to get into this state, and stays awake for more than two hours, can become almost impossible to settle.

In a situation like this sometimes a short period of 'crying down' has to be used as a last resort to solve the problem. This is the only situation where I would advise that young babies are left to cry for a short period, and even then it can only be done if you are confident that the baby has been well fed and winded.

Boredom

Even a newborn baby needs to be awake some of the time. Encourage him to be awake for a short spell after his day feeds. Babies under one month love to look at anything black and white such as a simple picture book. They also love pictures of faces, and the ones that fascinate them most will be the faces of their mummy and daddy. Try to divide toys into ones that are used for wakeful periods and ones that are used for winding-down time; bright, noisy toys for social time and calm, soothing toys for sleepy times.

Wind

All babies take a certain amount of wind while feeding, bottle-fed babies more so than breast-fed ones. Given the opportunity, most babies bring up their wind easily. If you suspect that your baby's crying is caused by wind, check that you are allowing enough time between feeds. I have found overfeeding and demand-feeding to be the main causes of colic in young babies. A breast-fed baby needs at least three hours to digest a full feed, and a formula-fed baby should be allowed three and a half to four hours. This time is always from the beginning of one feed to the beginning of the next feed.

I would also suggest that you keep a close eye on your baby's weight gain. If his weight gain is in excess of 240–300g (8–10oz) a week and he appears to be suffering from wind pains, it could be that he is overfeeding, particularly if he weighs over 3.6kg (8lb) and is feeding two or three times in the night. For details on how to deal with this problem refer to page 83.

Dummies

I have always believed that, if used with discretion, a dummy can be a great asset, especially for a sucky baby. However, I have always stressed the importance of never allowing the baby to have the dummy in his cot or allowing him to suck himself to sleep on the dummy. My advice was that it is fine to use it to calm a baby and, if necessary, settle him at sleep times, but it must be removed before he falls asleep. In my experience, allowing a baby to fall asleep with a dummy in his mouth is one of the worst sleep association problems to try to solve. He can end up waking several times a night, and each time he will expect the dummy to get back to sleep. That is why I always advised that the dummy is removed just before he drops off to sleep.

Since 2007, The Lullaby Trust has recommended the following advice on how the use of a dummy at all sleep times may help reduce the risk of cot death:

'Using a dummy every time you settle your baby to sleep – day and night – can reduce the risk of cot death. If breast-feeding, do not begin to give a dummy until your baby is one month old to ensure breast-feeding is well established. Don't worry if the dummy falls out while your baby is asleep, and don't force him to take a dummy if he doesn't want it. Never coat the dummy in anything sweet. Gradually wean him off a dummy after six months and before one year.'

In response to the advice from The Lullaby Trust, the UNICEF UK Friendly Initiative issued the following statement:

'While welcoming any research which may help to reduce the risk of sudden infant death syndrome (SIDS), there are considerations which must be taken into account before using this latest data to make recommendations to parents.

'Firstly, we must look at other research into dummies and SIDS. This tends to show that babies who used a dummy during their last sleep were less likely to die, but that routine dummy use is not protective. This may indicate that infants are at greater risk of SIDS if they routinely use a dummy but have not been given their dummy on a particular night.

'Secondly, the potential risks of dummy use need to be considered. These include:

- Interference with good establishment of breast-feeding in the early weeks.

- Increased risk of otitis media infection.

- Increased dental malocclusion.

- Risk of accidents such as obstruction of the airway.

'Thirdly, we need to ensure that the advice being proposed is realistic. If dummy use is really protective against SIDS but only if used every night, parents must be informed of this. The possibility that missing a night will increase risk among routine dummy users creates confusion and concern. We must be secure that parents will never forget to give the dummy once they have started to use it. It is therefore clear that we must support parents to make informed decisions about using a dummy, based on their own personal circumstances. This should include a discussion of the benefits and risks of dummy use, and acknowledgement that we do not know everything about the issue.'

If you have any concerns about the use of a dummy to reduce the risk of cot death, I would urge you to contact The Lullaby Trust directly so you can discuss the matter with them personally. When using the dummy at all sleep times during the first six months, it is possible that your baby will get into the habit of waking up several times a night looking for the dummy to be replaced. If this happens you will have to accept that when you start to eliminate the use of the dummy from six months, some form of sleep training will probably be needed to break the habit of your baby waking for the dummy. How best to eliminate the dummy after six months should be discussed with your health visitor. There are two types of dummy available: one has a round cherry-type teat, the other has a flat-shaped teat, which is called an orthodontic teat. Some experts claim that the orthodontic teat shape is better for the baby's mouth, but the problem with this type is that most young babies cannot hold them in for very long. I tend to use the cherry-type teat, and so far none of my babies appear to have developed an open bite, which is often the result of a dummy being used excessively once the teeth have come through. Whichever type of dummy you choose, buy several, thus allowing them to be changed frequently. The utmost attention should be paid to cleanliness when using a dummy; it should be washed and sterilised after each use. Never clean it by licking it, as so many parents do; there are more germs and bacteria in the mouth than you would believe.

Hiccups

Hiccups are very normal among tiny babies, and very few get distressed by them. Hiccups often happen after a feed. If it has been a night-time feed and your baby is due to go down for a sleep, it is advisable to go ahead and put him down regardless. If you wait until the hiccups are finished, there is a bigger chance of him falling asleep in your arms, which is something to be avoided at all costs. If your baby is one of the rare ones who gets upset by their hiccups, then try giving him the recommended dose of gripe water, which can sometimes help.

Possetting

It is very common for some babies to bring up a small amount of milk while being burped or after a feed. It is called possetting, and for most babies it does not create a problem. However, if your baby is regularly gaining more than 240g (8oz) of weight each week it could be that he is drinking too much. With a bottle-fed baby the problem is easily solved as you are able to see how much the baby is drinking and therefore slightly reduce the amount at the feeds during which he appears to possett more. It is more difficult to tell how much a breast-fed baby is drinking. But by keeping a note of which feeds cause more possetting, and reducing the time on the breast at those feeds, the possetting may be reduced. If your baby is possetting excessively and not gaining weight it could be that he is suffering from a condition called 'reflux' (see below). With babies who are inclined to bring up milk, it is important to keep them as upright as possible after a feed, and special care should be taken when burping.

Top Tips

Any baby bringing up an entire feed twice in a row should be seen by a doctor immediately.

Reflux

Sometimes a baby displaying all the symptoms of colic (see page 293) actually has a condition called gastro-oesophageal reflux disease (GORD). Babies often bring up a small amount of milk after a feed and this is known as 'posseting' (see above) or 'reflux'. Many babies experience a small amount of reflux at some point in their first year as the muscle at the lower end of the oesophagus is too weak to keep the milk in the baby's stomach, so it comes back up, along with acid from the stomach, causing a very painful burning sensation in the oesophagus. However, excessive posseting is one of the symptoms of GORD, a more long-term and serious form of reflux. If your baby is arching his back during feeding, refusing to feed and crying, posseting excessively or coughing a lot at night, he may be suffering from GORD. In some cases, not all babies with reflux actually sick up the milk, and suffer from what the medical profession call 'silent reflux'.

These babies can often be misdiagnosed as having colic. They can be very difficult to feed, constantly arching their backs and screaming during a feed. They also tend to get very irritable when laid flat, and no amount of cuddling or rocking will calm them when they are like this.

If your baby displays these symptoms, ask your GP to refer your baby to a specialist paediatrician. I have seen too many cases of babies being diagnosed as having colic, when in fact they were suffering from reflux, despite not being sick. If you think that your baby is suffering from reflux, it is essential that you do not allow anyone to dismiss the pains as colic. Reflux is very stressful for the baby and parents, and it is essential that you get ongoing advice and support from your GP and health visitor.

If you feel that you are not getting the help you need, do not be frightened to ask for a second opinion. If reflux is not the problem, you will at least have eliminated it as a possible cause. If it is the problem, with the help of the right medication, your baby will have been saved months of misery from the pain it can cause.

It is recommended that babies with reflux are fed little and often and kept upright for at least 30 minutes after feeding. However, while keeping a baby upright after feeding for 30 minutes can certainly help with reflux, it can sometimes lead to other problems. For example, if your baby is ready to sleep fairly soon after he is fed, it is inevitable that he will fall asleep on your shoulder. If he then wakes up immediately or very soon after you transfer him to his bed, you will have to spend a considerable time trying to resettle an upset, possibly overtired baby.

To avoid a sleep association problem arising because the baby is falling asleep on you, I would recommend that you try to structure your baby's feeding so that whenever possible he is not ready for a sleep immediately after feeds. The following feeding and sleeping schedule for a baby under six months will ensure that for most of the time he is not due to sleep immediately after feeding. Obviously, you will need to adjust it to suit your baby's individual needs which are dependent on age, but following a plan like this or similar will ensure that settling problems are less likely:

7.00am	awake and feeding
7.30am	holding upright
8.00am	social time
8.30–9am	nap time
10.00am	awake
10.15–10.30am	feeding
11.00am	holding time
11.30am	short play and cuddle time
11.45am	nap time
2.00pm	awake time
2.15–2.30pm	feeding
3.00pm	holding time
4–4.30pm	nap time
5.00pm	split feed
5.30pm	holding time
6.00pm	bath
6.15pm	small settling bedtime feed

6.30pm	holding time
6.45pm	settling time
7.00pm	sleep time
10.00pm	awake and feeding
10.30pm	holding time
11.15pm	offer remainder of feed
11.30pm	settling time

In the night I would recommend that you follow the same approach as the late feed. I usually find that because babies are more sleepy at the middle of the night feed, they are more relaxed and can be settled back to sleep with less holding time. I would also recommend that at all times you put loose clothing on your baby. While trendy little jeans or leggings look cute, any clothing with a waist band can cause discomfort to babies after they have been fed.

I have discovered that once a baby is on the correct medication then I can usually reduce the time they are kept upright to between 10 and 15 minutes. I have also found that positioning cushions under my left arm, then holding the baby on a pillow at a 30–40 degree slope whilst feeding and for 10–15 minutes after being burped, really worked well and was not as tiring as holding him totally upright. If you have a chair with a 30 degree slope that keeps your baby's back totally straight, it may be worthwhile trying it out. Car seats and most regular baby seats should be avoided as they do not allow the baby's body to remain straight enough.

Some babies may need medication for several months until the muscles tighten up. Fortunately, the majority of babies outgrow the condition by the time they are one year old. If your baby is diagnosed with reflux it is worth taking a look at the reflux section on my website contentedbaby.com. Here you will find case studies, plus lots of advice and tips on how to survive those early months with a reflux baby.

Separation anxiety

At around the age of six months babies start to gain more understanding of their environment and begin to realise that they are separate from their mothers. Between the ages of six and twelve months most babies may show some signs of separation anxiety. You may find that your happy contented baby, who was so easy-going and relaxed, suddenly becomes clingy, anxious and demanding, and might start crying the minute you leave the room. This sudden change of your baby's temperament can be very upsetting to deal with, but do be reassured that this behaviour is a totally normal part of a baby's development. Most babies will go through this stage to some degree.

Although this stage can be a very exhausting time for you, it rarely lasts long. The following guidelines can help make this difficult period less stressful:

• If you are planning to return to work when your baby is between six months and one year, try to make sure that he gets accustomed to being left with someone else before he reaches six months. If you are the sole carer, and he is not used to any other person looking after him for the majority of his day, it is more likely that he will find a prolonged separation upsetting. Think about arrangements that can work for you. If you are able to afford a little child care it would be good to organise your weekly routine so that he spends some time with a childminder, even if it is only a couple of hours a week. Alternately, arrange with a friend a time when you look after each other's children. It is really helpful for your baby to begin to understand that you can leave and return. This minimises any anxiety, not just for you but also for your baby.

• Aim to get your baby used to the nursery or childminder at least one month before returning to work. Gradually lengthen the period of time you leave him. If your childminder is able to support you with this it will make the more prolonged absences easier for you both.

- The longer you give yourself and your child the time to get used to separation, the more flexibility it will give you. For instance, if your baby is inconsolable about your departure you could delay trying to leave him again for a week or so. With such a young child, every day adds to his confidence and understanding, and it might be that if you leave it for a week or so, your baby has a different response next time you try to leave him.

- If your baby has a particular activity he enjoys – hitting a saucepan with a spoon, or playing with a particular toy – try to organise for your baby's childminder or carer to have something similar to offer.

- Use roleplay as a way of helping your baby understand about people leaving and returning. Place a dolly or a teddy in a different room to where your child normally is during the day. By visiting the room on a regular basis and saying hello and goodbye to the toys will help him understand the concept.

- Praise your baby when he is prepared to go with your friend or childminder.

- Talk to your baby. It is extraordinary how much a little baby can take in. If your baby is used to his father leaving for work each day, try if possible to be with your baby when your partner leaves so that you can wave him off together. Keep repeating: 'Daddy has gone to work'. This will reinforce his confidence that when the time comes for Mummy to go to work, you will be returning.

- When the time comes for you to leave your baby, make sure that you keep your goodbyes to a minimum. Be positive, use reassuring phrases and smile; this will help to reassure your baby. Always give your baby a hug, kiss and a wave when you leave him, along with a verbal reminder that you will be back soon. Using the same approach and words each time you say goodbye will, in the long term, be more reassuring than going back to try to calm him down. While a baby will often cry when a mother or main carer leaves the room, most children will be easy to distract in the hands of a competent carer. However babies are sensitive to moods, and if you are anxious and worried your baby will pick up on this and be more likely to be upset.

- It also helps when you finish an activity with your baby to say 'Bye, bye' to his toys, his bed, the television etc., as this helps to reinforce that whenever he leaves something or someone he will see them again.

- Try to avoid just slipping away when you leave your baby. Although you will find it difficult if he is upset when you say goodbye, it is much better for him to understand that you are going and that you will return, rather than simply slipping away and for him to look around later to find that you have vanished. This could contribute to his unhappiness – he might become confused and clingy for fear of you just vanishing.

- Be realistic – you might well find that your baby is fretful at home even though the carer has told you that he is happy and content when you are not there. In the same way that you will find the change to your routine tiring, so will your baby. Don't worry; providing that the circumstances are loving and secure, babies are adaptable.

- During this period of adjustment ask your baby's carer to ensure that your baby is not subjected to too many new experiences or for him to be handled by strangers. The calmer and more predictable his routine, the quicker he will get over his feelings of anxiety.

- If your baby is used to just being with you for the first six months, you can imagine that adapting to a livelier environment can be challenging. If you have chosen a childminder who looks after other children or a nanny share, your baby will need to adapt to a noisier, more dynamic environment than he is used to. You can help your baby by arranging regular play dates with only a small group of mothers and babies. Not only will this be enjoyable for you, but it will also enable your baby to get used to the noise and activity of other children. If you have a nervous baby you will find that he will become happier once he is used to a different environment. Gradually introduce him into larger groups and other experiences. Generally babies love the activities of toddlers so, providing that they are appropriately monitored, you can feel reassured that it will be a pleasant experience for him.

Stranger anxiety

At around six months you might also find that your sociable baby is much more wary of strangers. This is a natural part of his development. There is a theory that this fear of strangers is a biological response relating to our origins. A fear of strangers was a natural protective response that contributed to a baby's ability to survive in a primitive environment.

We have an expectation that babies are happy to be handed to loving relatives and friends for cuddles when they are small, but even small babies can find being passed from one loving relative to the next is tiring and at times distressing.

- If your baby begins to cry when approached by strangers, or to look away when someone is trying to engage them, don't attempt to push them to communicate. It is much better to explain that your child is becoming self-conscious and having a shy period than to expect your baby to smile on cue.

- You can ease this response to those friends and family you see regularly by talking to your baby about them. You can show your baby photographs and explain who they are.

- For those grandparents or family who see your baby occasionally it can be upsetting when your baby is distressed or tearful, but be reassured that any initial concern will not last long if you are all in a position to spend some time together.

- Role play can also help in this circumstance; try giving your baby's toys the names of the friends and family who you want him to be familiar with.

- Consider explaining to friends not to make too much fuss of your baby on first arrival. Sometimes a baby can find their physical proximity threatening, and it is easier if the baby is allowed to respond in his own time, when he feels comfortable with the new arrival, rather than when someone is attempting to make eye contact and communicate.

- Although your baby will learn how to deal with greetings and attention as he grows up, some children remain shy. It is much better for you to adapt to this and try to understand how it feels to be a shy child, rather than pushing your child into situations where they feel uncomfortable or distressed.

Common feeding problems

Difficult feeder

The majority of newborn babies take to the breast or bottle quickly and easily. Unlike the new mother, who has much to learn about feeding, the baby usually instinctively knows what is expected of him. However, there are some babies who, from day one, will fuss and fret within minutes of being put on the breast or being offered the bottle. I often find that some babies who have undergone a particularly hard birth can be more difficult to feed.

If you find that your baby becomes tense and fretful at feed times, try to avoid having visitors then. No matter how well-meaning family and friends may be, it will be impossible to keep things completely calm and quiet if you are having to make conversation. The following guidelines, regardless of whether you are breast- or bottle-feeding, should help make feeding a tense baby easier:

- It is essential that the handling of tense babies is kept to the minimum. Avoid overstimulation and handing the baby from person to person, especially before a feed.

- Whenever possible, try to give the feed in a quiet room with a calm atmosphere. Apart from perhaps one person to offer practical help and emotional support, no other person should be allowed in the room.

- Prepare everything needed for the feed well in advance. Try and make sure that you have rested and have eaten.

- Avoid turning on the television during a feed, put your phone on silent and in another room, and play some calm music.

- When the baby wakes for his feed, delay changing his nappy as this may trigger crying.

- Try swaddling him firmly in a soft cotton sheet to prevent him thrashing his arms and legs around. Make sure that you are comfortable before you start feeding.

- Do not attempt to latch the baby on to the breast or put the bottle straight in his mouth if he is crying. Hold him firmly in the feeding position and calm him down with continuous gentle patting on the back.

- Try holding a dummy in his mouth. Once he has calmed down and has sucked steadily for a few minutes, then very quickly ease the dummy out and offer him the breast or the bottle.

If you find your baby is fussy when feeding and taking a lot longer than an hour to feed, try allowing him a short break mid-way during the feed. It is better to let your baby feed in two shorter spurts than spend a lengthy time trying to force your baby to feed. If your baby has been feeding well and suddenly starts to refuse the breast or bottle, it could be because he is feeling unwell. Ear infections can easily go undetected and are a very common cause of a baby not wanting to feed. If your baby shows any of the following signs it would be advisable to consult your doctor:

- Sudden loss of appetite, and becoming upset when offered a feed.

- Disruption to the normal sleep pattern.

- Suddenly becoming clingy and whingey.

- Becomes lethargic and unsociable.

Low milk supply

As they grow, all babies will increase the amount they drink. However, the feeds must be structured to co-ordinate with the baby's growth, thereby encouraging him to take more milk at individual feeds. If not, he will be very likely to continue to feed little and often.

All too often, I get calls from the parents of older babies who are still following the demand rules of milk feeding. While the majority of these babies are over 12 weeks and are physically capable of drinking more at individual feeds, they continue to feed as they did as newborns – often 8–10 times a day. Many breast-fed babies are still having only one breast at each feed, while bottle-fed babies may only be taking 90–120ml (3–4oz) of formula. In order to go for longer spells between feeds, the majority of babies should be taking from both breasts at each feed, or have a formula feed of 210–240ml (7–8oz). It is my firm belief that it is during those early days of milk feeding that the foundation is laid for healthy eating habits in the future. To avoid long-term feeding problems that can affect your baby's sleep, it is advisable to structure and solve any milk-feeding problems early on. Not producing enough milk, especially later in the day, is a very common problem for breast-feeding mothers and one of the major reasons breast-feeding goes wrong. I believe that hunger is why so many babies are fretful and difficult to settle in the evening. If the problem of a low milk supply is not resolved in the early days, then a pattern soon emerges of the baby needing to feed on and off all evening to try and satisfy his needs. Mothers are advised that this constant feeding is normal and the best way to increase the milk supply, but in my experience, it usually has the opposite effect. Because the amount of milk the breasts produce is dictated by the amount of milk the baby drinks, these frequent feeds signal the breasts to produce milk little and often. These small feeds will rarely satisfy the baby, leaving him hungry and irritable. I believe that the stress involved in frequently feeding a very hungry, irritable and often overtired baby can cause many mothers to become so exhausted that their milk supply is reduced even further. A low milk supply and exhaustion go hand-in-hand. I am convinced that by expressing a small amount of milk during the early weeks of breast-feeding, when the breasts are producing more milk than the baby needs, the mother can help avoid the problem of a low milk supply.

If your baby is under one month of age and not settling in the evening, it is possible the cause is a low milk supply. Expressing at the times suggested in the routine below should help solve this problem. The short amount of time you spend expressing will ensure that during any future growth spurts you will be producing enough milk to meet any increase in your baby's appetite. If your baby is over one month and not settling in the evening or after daytime feeds, the following six-day plan will quickly help to increase your milk supply. The temporary introduction of top-up feeds will ensure that your baby is not subjected to hours of irritability and anxiety caused by hunger, which is what usually happens when mothers resort to demand-feeding to increase their milk supply.

Plan for increased milk supply

Days one to three

6.45am

- Express 30ml (1oz) from each breast.

- Baby should be awake, and feeding no later than 7am, regardless of how often he fed in the night.

- He should be offered up to 20–25 minutes on the fullest breast, then up to 10–15 minutes on the second breast.

- Do not feed after 7.45am. He can stay awake for up to two hours.

8am

- It is very important that you have breakfast and a drink no later than 8am.

9am

- If your baby has not been settling well for his nap, offer him up to 5–10 minutes on the breast from which he last fed.

- Try to have a short rest when the baby is sleeping.

10am

- Baby must be fully awake now, regardless of how long he slept.

- He should be given up to 20–25 minutes from the breast he last fed on while you drink a glass of water and have a small snack.

- Express 60ml (2oz) from the second breast, then offer him up to 10–20 minutes on the same breast.

11.45am

- He should be given the 60ml (2oz) that you expressed to ensure that he does not wake up hungry during his midday nap.

- It Is very important that you have a good lunch and a rest before the next feed.

2pm

- Baby should be awake and feeding no later than 2pm, regardless of how long he has slept.

- Give him up to 20–25 minutes from the breast he last fed on while you drink a glass of water. Express 60ml (2oz) from the second breast, then offer up to 10–20 minutes on the same breast.

4pm

- Baby will need a short nap according to the routine appropriate for his age.

5pm

- Baby should be fully awake and feeding no later than 5pm.

- Give up to 15–20 minutes from both breasts.

6.15pm

- Baby should be offered a top-up feed of expressed milk from the bottle. A baby under 3.6kg (8lb) in weight will probably settle with 60–90ml (2–3oz); bigger babies may need 120–150ml (4–5oz).

- Once your baby is settled, it is important that you have a good meal and a rest.

8pm

- Express from both breasts.

10pm

- It is important that you express from both breasts at this time, as the amount you get will be a good indicator of how much milk you are producing.

- Arrange for your partner or another family member to give the late feed to the baby so you can have an early night.

10.30pm

- Baby should be awake and feeding no later than 10.30pm. He can be given a full feed of either formula or expressed milk from a bottle. Refer to page 73–5 for details of the amounts to give.

In the night

- A baby who has had a full feed from the bottle at 10.30pm should manage to get to 2–2.30am. He should then be offered upto 20–25 minutes from the first breast, then 10–15 minutes from the second. In order to avoid a second waking in the night at 5am, it is very important that he feeds from both breasts.

If your baby fed well at 10.30pm and wakes earlier than 2am, the cause may not be hunger. Other reasons which may be causing him to wake earlier could be kicking off the covers or your baby not being fully awake at the late feed. A baby under six weeks who wakes up thrashing around may still need to be fully swaddled. A baby over six weeks may benefit from being half-swaddled under the arms in a thin cotton sheet. With all babies, it is important to ensure that the top sheet is tucked in well, down the sides and at the bottom of the cot, pushing at least six inches of the sheet under the mattress. Refer to pages 6–7 or www.contentedbaby.com on how to make up the cot properly.

With a baby who is waking up before 2am, it may be worthwhile keeping him awake longer, and offering him some more milk just before you settle him at around 11.15pm. See page 107 for information on how doing a split, late feed can help a baby sleep longer in the night.

Day four

By day four, your breasts should be feeling fuller in the morning and the following alterations should be made to the above plan:

- If your baby is sleeping well between 9–9.45am, reduce the time on the breast at 9am to five minutes.

- The top-up at 11.45am can be reduced by 30ml (1oz) if he is sleeping well at lunchtime, or shows signs of not feeding so well at the 2pm feed.

- The expressing at the 2pm feed should be dropped, which should mean that your breasts are fuller by the 5pm feed.

- If you feel your breasts are fuller at 5pm, make sure he totally empties the first breast before putting him on to the second breast. If he has not emptied the second breast before his bath, he should be offered it again after the bath, and before he is given a top-up.

- The 8pm expressing should be dropped and the 10pm expressing brought forward to 9.30pm. It is important that both breasts are completely emptied at the 9.30pm expressing.

Day five

- Dropping the 2pm and 8pm expressing on the fourth day should result in your breasts being very engorged on the morning of the fifth day; it is very important that the extra milk is totally emptied at the first feed in the morning.

- At the 7am feed the baby should be offered up to 20–25 minutes on the fullest breast, then up to 10–15 minutes on the second breast, after you have expressed. The amount you express will depend on the weight of your baby. It is important that you take just the right amount so that enough is left for your baby to get a full feed. If you managed to express a minimum of 120ml (4oz) at the late feed, you should manage to express the following amounts:

(a) Baby weighing 3.6–4.5kg (8–10lb) – express 120ml (4oz)

(b) Baby weighing 4.5–5.4kg (10–12lb) – express 90ml (3oz)

(c) Baby weighing over 5.4kg (12lb) – express 60ml (2oz)

Day six

- By the sixth day, your milk supply should have increased enough for you to drop all top-up feeds, and follow the breast-feeding routines appropriate for your baby's age.

It is very important that you also follow the guidelines for expressing as set out in the routines. This will ensure that you will be able to satisfy your baby's increased appetite during his next growth spurt. I would also suggest that you continue with one bottle of either expressed or formula milk at the late feed until your baby is weaned on to solids at six months. This will allow the feed to be given by your husband or partner, enabling you to get to bed earlier after you have expressed, which, in turn, will make it easier for you to cope with the middle-of-the-night feed.

Excessive night feeding

I have found that all babies, even demand-fed babies, are capable of sleeping one longer spell between feeds by the time they reach 4–6 weeks of age. Beatrice Hollyer and Lucy Smith, authors of an excellent book called *Sleep: The Secret of Problem-free Nights*, describe this longer stretch of sleep as the 'core night' and I have referred to it on page 322. They advise parents to take their cue from this, which they believe is the foundation of encouraging a baby to sleep right through the night.

I believe that by the end of the second week a baby who weighed 2.1kg (7lb) or more at birth should really only need one feed in the night (between midnight and 6am). This is provided, of course, that he is feeding well at all of his daytime feeds and gets a full feed between 10–11pm. In my experience, regardless of whether he is breast- or bottle-fed, a baby who continues to feed two or three times in the night will eventually begin to cut back on his daytime feeds. A vicious circle soon emerges, where the baby ends up genuinely needing to feed in the night so that his daily nutritional needs can be met.

With bottle-fed babies it is easier to avoid a pattern of excessive night-time feeding evolving by monitoring the amounts they are getting during the day. Calculate how much milk your baby needs each day for his weight. Then use the example chart on page 75 to see how to structure feeds, so the biggest feeds are at the night times. This, as well as the core night suggestions (page 322), will prevent excessive night-feeding for a formula-fed baby. Excessive night-time feeding is considered normal for breast-fed babies and is actually encouraged by many breast-feeding experts. Mothers are advised to have their baby sleep with them, so that he can feed on and off throughout the night. Much emphasis is placed on the fact that the hormone prolactin, which is necessary for making breast milk, is produced more at night. The theory is that mothers who feed their babies more in the night than in the day are much more likely to sustain a good milk supply. This advice obviously works for some mothers, but breast-feeding statistics prove that it clearly doesn't for many others, as so many give up in the first month. As I've said, I believe that the exhaustion caused by so many night-time feeds is one of the main reasons that so many mothers give up breast-feeding. In my experience from working with hundreds of breast-feeding mothers, I have found that a good stretch of sleep in the night results in the breasts producing more milk.

A full and satisfying feed in the middle of the night will ensure that the baby settles back to sleep quickly until the morning.

The following guidelines give the main causes of excessive night-time feeding and how it can be avoided:

- A premature baby or a very tiny baby may need to feed more often than three-hourly, and medical advice should be sought on how best to deal with these special circumstances.

- If he feeds well at every feed (a baby over 3.6kg/8lb should always be offered the second breast) and is sleeping well at all the other sleep times, he may not be getting enough from the late feed.

- If a low milk supply at the last feed is the problem, it can easily be solved by ensuring your baby takes a full feed from a bottle of either formula or expressed milk. If you decide to offer expressed milk, you will need to allow enough time to express for the feed, which can be added to milk from the morning expressing.

- Many women are concerned that introducing a bottle too early may reduce the baby's desire to take the breast. All of my babies were offered one bottle a day as a matter of course and I have never had one baby who had nipple confusion or refused the breast. It has the added advantage that the father can give the last feed and enable the mother to get to bed by 10pm.

- If after one week of giving a full feed at this time there is no improvement, and your baby is still waking several times a night, it is more likely that your baby has a problem with his sleeping than with his feeding. I suggest that you continue to offer the bottle for a further week and refer to page 342 for more advice on night waking.

- Babies under 3.6kg (8lb) in weight who are changed to the second breast before they reach the fatty, rich hind milk in the first breast will be more likely to wake more than once in the night.

- If a baby weighs over 3.6kg (8lb) in weight at birth and is only feeding from one breast at a feed, then he may not be getting enough milk, and should be offered the second breast at some or all of his feeds. If he has fed for 20–25 minutes on the first breast then try to get him to take 5–10 minutes from the second. If he refuses, try waiting 15–20 minutes before offering it again.

The majority of the babies on my routines who are only feeding once in the night gradually push themselves right through the night, dropping the middle-of-the-night feed as soon as they are physically capable. However, occasionally I get a baby who reaches six weeks and continues to wake at 2am looking for a feed. In my experience, allowing these babies to continue to feed at this time usually results in them reducing the amount they take at 7am, often cutting this feed out altogether. When this happens, I would use the core night method below to ensure that when the baby is ready to reduce the number of feeds he is having over a 24-hour period, it is always the middle-of-the-night feed that he drops first.

The core night method

The core night method has been used for many years by maternity nurses and parents who believe in routine. It works on the principle that once a baby sleeps for one longer spell in the night, he should never again be fed during the hours slept in the course of the core night. If he wakes during those hours, he should be left for a few minutes to settle himself back to sleep. If he refuses to settle, then other methods apart from feeding should be used to settle him. Hollyer and Smith recommend patting, offering a dummy or giving a sip of water. However, I must stress that it is now recommended that babies under six months are not given water. Please refer to page 83 about giving water to very young babies. Attention should be kept to the minimum while reassuring the baby that you are there. They claim that following this approach will, within days, have your baby sleeping at least the hours of his first core night. It also teaches the baby the most important two sleep skills: how to go to sleep, and how to go back to sleep after surfacing from a non-REM (rapid eye movement) sleep. Dr Brian Symon, author of *Silent Nights* and a senior lecturer in general practice at the University of Adelaide, recommends a similar approach for babies over six weeks. For babies who are putting on a good amount of weight each week, but who are still waking at 3am, if the baby refuses to settle then give the shortest feed possible that will allow him to settle.

Before embarking on these methods, the following points should be read carefully to make sure that your baby really is capable of going for a longer spell in the night:

- These methods should never be used with a very small baby or a baby who is not gaining weight. A baby not gaining weight should always be seen by a doctor.

- The above methods should only be used if your baby is gaining weight steadily, and if you are sure that his last feed is substantial enough to help him sleep for the longer stretch in the night.

- The main sign that a baby is ready to cut down on a night feed is a regular weight gain and the reluctance to feed, or tendency to feed less, at 7am.

- The aim of using any of the above methods is gradually to increase the length of time your baby can go from his last feed and not to eliminate the night feed in one go.

- The core night method can be used if, over three or four nights, a baby has shown signs that he is capable of sleeping for a longer stretch.

- If your baby does not settle within 20 minutes of using the core night method, then he should be given a big enough feed to get him through to nearer 7am. There is no advantage to having your baby awake for lengthy periods in the night, as it will only cause him to need more sleep during the day. Too much sleep in the day will only cause him to be more unsettled in the night.

- It can be used to try and reduce the number of times a demand-fed baby is fed in the night and to encourage him to go for a longer stretch between feeds, or after his last daytime feed.

Sleepy feeder

Sometimes a very sleepy baby may be inclined to keep dozing during the feed, but if he does not want to take the required amount he will end up wanting to feed again in an hour or two. This is a good time to change his nappy, burp him and encourage him to finish his feed. Making a little effort in the early days to keep your baby awake enough to drink the correct amount at each feed, and at the times given in the routine, will in the long term be well worthwhile. Some babies will take half the feed, have a stretch and kick for 10–15 minutes, and then be happy to take the rest. The important thing that I have found with sleepy babies is not to force them to stay awake by talking too much or jiggling them about. By putting your baby on the play mat and leaving him for 10 minutes, you will probably find that he will get enough of a second wind to take more of a feed. During the first months, allow up to 45 minutes to one hour for a feed.

Obviously, if he does not feed well at a particular feed, and wakes early from his sleep, he must be fed. Do not attempt to try and stretch him to the next feed, otherwise he will be so tired that the next feed will also become another sleepy feed. Top him up and treat the feed like a night feed, and try to settle him back to sleep so that you can get his feeding back on track for the evening.

Another technique that can be used to solve a range of breast-feeding problems, including sleepy feeding, is 'skin-to-skin contact'. We know that babies love to be cuddled and held, but research shows that contact with their mother's skin does more than just make them happy. It is thought skin-to-skin contact stimulates a part of the baby's brain that prompts a desire to seek nourishment in order to continue developing. The pressure of the direct contact with his mother also gives the baby a sense of safety so he will be happier to feed. In contrast, a baby who is sleeping on the breast, may in fact be in 'shut down' mode because he is stressed and attempts to wake him to feed him only add to that stress. Putting a baby into skin-to-skin contact will therefore not only alert a sleepy baby but calm an over-stimulated or stressed one.

Over the years I have picked up other tips and techniques on how to get a sleepy baby to feed well, from working with premature babies and babies in special care:

- Make sure that your baby is fully awake before starting a feed. Changing his nappy and wiping his face and hands with a damp facecloth will help get the baby properly awake before feeding.

- During the day feed him in a bright room; place a change mat on the floor right next to the chair where you are feeding.

- Try to wear a cool, short-sleeved t-shirt or blouse instead of a warm woolly long–sleeved sweater, which would give the baby the feeling of being enclosed in a blanket while feeding and encourage the baby to feel sleepy.

- Undo the legs of his babygrow, so that his legs are fully exposed to the air. With a very sleepy baby, strip him down to his vest.

- With breast-fed babies, during the feed massage their feet, stroke their face, and with your forefinger and middle finger gently press upwards on their chin when they stop sucking.

- With bottle-fed babies who stop sucking during the feed, moving the teat around in their mouth will often get them sucking again. I also found that holding the bottle around the neck with my thumb, forefinger and middle finger, instead of midway down the bottle, meant that I could use my remaining fingers to gently press upwards on their chin to get them feeding again.

- If despite doing all of the above they were either falling asleep on the feed, or feeding for more than a minute or so with their eyes closed, I would gently remove them from the breast or bottle and place them flat on the changing mat for a minute or so. Sometimes I would have to do this several times during a feed, but I found that the perseverance was worth it, as within a week or so the babies had learned to stay awake well during feeds and also happily for a short spell after feeds. This meant that as well as taking a full feed, they would then sleep much better and longer for both daytime naps and night-time sleep.

Refusal of milk

The amount of milk a six-month-old baby drinks will gradually begin to reduce as his intake of solid food increases. However, up to the age of nine months, a baby still needs a minimum of 500–600ml (18–20oz) a day of breast or formula milk. This daily amount gradually reduces to a minimum of 350ml (12oz) at one year of age. If your baby is losing interest or refusing some of his milk feeds and taking less than the recommended amounts, careful attention should be given to the timing of solids and the type of food given.

With breast-fed babies it is impossible to know exactly what they are getting but the following advice will hopefully help determine some possible causes of why he is refusing milk feeds:

- At the age of six months, a baby should still be taking 4–5 full milk feeds during the day between 6–7am and 10–11pm. A full milk feed consists of 210–240ml (7–8oz) or a feed from both breasts. Babies under six months who are weaned early on the advice of a health visitor or GP should not be given solids in the middle of their milk feed. They will be more likely to refuse the remainder of their formula or the second breast. Give most of the milk feed first, then the solids.

- A baby under six months of age still needs a full milk feed at 11am. If he is being weaned early on medical advice, introducing breakfast too soon or offering too much solid food before his 11am milk feed could cause him to reduce the amount of milk he takes too quickly, or refuse the milk feed altogether.

- The 11am milk feed should be reduced and eliminated between the ages of six and seven months. If you started weaning earlier than six months, it is possible that by six months your baby will only be drinking a small amount of milk, and once protein is introduced the lunch time milk feed can be dropped, which should help increase his appetite for solids.

- Giving lunchtime solids at 2pm and evening solids at 5pm is the reason many babies under seven months cut down too quickly or refuse their 6pm milk feed. Until he is used to solids, it is better to give a baby his lunchtime solids at 11am and his evening solids after he has had some milk at 5pm.

- Giving foods that take longer to digest such as banana or avocado at the wrong time of the day can cause a baby to cut back on the next milk feed. You should pay special attention when introducing new foods. Until a baby reaches seven months, it is better to serve these types of food after the 6pm feed, rather than during the day.

- Babies over six months of age who begin to refuse milk are often being allowed too many snacks in between meals or too much juice. Try replacing juice with water and cutting out snacks in between meals.

- Between nine and twelve months, some babies begin refusing the bedtime milk feed, which is a sign that they are ready to drop their third milk feed. If this happens, it is important to reduce the amount given at the 2.30pm feed, before eventually dropping it altogether.

Refusal of solids

With babies of six months or older, the refusal of solids often occurs because they drink too much milk, especially if they are still feeding in the middle of the night. Every day I speak to parents of babies and toddlers who will barely touch solids, let alone eat three meals a day. In the majority of these cases, the babies are still being milk-fed on demand, some feeding as often as two or three times in the night. While milk is still a very important food for babies at six months, failing to structure the time of milk feeds and the amounts given can seriously affect the introduction of solids. If your baby is refusing solids, the following guidelines will help you determine the cause:

- The recommended age to introduce solids is at six months. If your baby is six months and sleeping through the night from 10pm this feed should gradually be reduced and eliminated. Refer to pages 240–248 on how to do this.

- A baby is ready to be weaned when he shows signs that his appetite is no longer satisfied with 4–5 full milk feeds a day. A full milk feed is either a formula-feed of 240ml (8oz) or a feed from both breasts. See page 245 for signs that your baby is ready for weaning.

- If your baby reaches six months and is having more than 4–5 full milk feeds a day, his refusal of solids may be caused by drinking too much milk. It is important to cut right back on his 11am milk feed to encourage him to eat more solids at that time. By the end of six months, a baby's milk intake should be a minimum of 600ml (20oz) a day, divided between three drinks a day and small amounts used in food. If your baby is still refusing solids at this age, despite cutting down on his milk intake, it is important that you discuss the problem as soon as possible with your doctor or health visitor.

Fussy feeder

If milk feeding is structured properly during the early days of weaning, the majority of babies will happily eat most of the foods they are offered. By the time they reach nine months, babies are expected to be getting most of their nourishment from eating three solid meals a day. Parents are advised to offer their babies a wide variety of foods to ensure they receive all the nutrients they need. However, it is often around this time that many babies start to reject food they have previously enjoyed. If your baby is between nine and twelve months of age and suddenly starts to reject his food, or becomes fussy and fretful at meal times, the following guidelines should help determine the cause:

- Parents often have unrealistic expectations of the amounts of food their baby should have, and serving too large portions can mislead them into thinking that their baby has a feeding problem. The following list, showing the amounts of food a baby aged between nine and twelve months of age needs, will help you decide if your baby is eating enough solids:

    a. 3–4 servings of carbohydrate, made up of cereal, whole-meal bread, pasta or potatoes. A serving is one slice of bread, 30g (1oz) of cereal, two tablespoonfuls of pasta, or a small baked potato.

    b. 3–4 portions of vegetables and fruit, including raw vegetables. A portion is one small apple, pear or banana, carrot, a couple of cauliflower or broccoli florets, or two tablespoons of chopped green beans.

    c. One portion of animal protein or vegetable protein. A portion is 30g (1oz) of poultry, meat or fish, or 60g (2oz) of lentil and pulses.

- Self-feeding plays an important role in a baby's mental and physical development as it encourages hand-eye co-ordination and increases his sense of independence. Between six and nine months of age, most babies will start to pick up their food and try to feed themselves. The whole business of feeding can become very messy and mealtimes take much longer. Restricting a baby's natural desire to explore his food and feed himself will only lead to frustration and, very often, refusal to be spoon-fed. Introducing lots of finger foods and allowing him to eat part of his meal by himself, regardless of the mess he makes, will make him much more inclined to take the remainder from you from a spoon.

- By the time a baby reaches nine months of age, he will become more interested in the colour, shape and texture of his food. A baby who is still having all the different foods mashed up together will quickly begin to get bored with even his favourite foods and this is one of the main reasons that babies lose interest in vegetables.

- Offering your baby a selection of vegetables of various textures and colours at each meal in small amounts will be more appealing to him than a large amount of just one or two vegetables mashed together.

- Sweet puddings and desserts served on a regular basis are major causes of babies and toddlers refusing their main course. Even babies as young as nine months can quickly learn that if they refuse the savoury foods and fuss enough, they will more than likely be given pudding. It is better to restrict puddings and desserts to special occasions, and serve your baby chopped vegtables, cheese with rice cakes/breadsticks or yoghurt.

- If your baby rejects a particular food, it is important that he should be offered it again a couple of weeks later. Babies' likes and dislikes regarding food fluctuate a good deal in the first year and parents who fail to keep reintroducing food that is rejected usually find that their baby ends up eating a very restricted diet.

- Giving large amounts of juice or water prior to a meal can result in a baby not eating very well. Try to offer him drinks midway between meals, not an hour before. Also, at mealtimes encourage him to eat at least half of the solids before offering him a drink of water.

- The timing of meals also plays a big part in how well a baby eats. A baby who is having his breakfast solids much later than 8am is unlikely to be very hungry for his lunch much before 1pm. Likewise, a baby who is having teatime solids later than 5pm may be getting too tired to eat well.

- Try to aim to have your baby consume breakfast milk and solids between 7am and 8am, so that he is hungry for his lunch around 12–12.15pm, so that there is a big enough gap between lunch and tea.

- Giving too many snacks in between meals can often take the edge off a baby's appetite. Try restricting snacks for a couple of days to see if his appetite improves at mealtimes.

If you are concerned that your baby is not taking enough solids, it is advisable to seek advice from your health visitor or doctor. Keeping a diary for a week, listing the times and amounts of all food and drinks consumed, will help them to determine the cause of your baby's feeding problems.

Tongue tie

Tongue tie is a condition in which the tissue which attaches a baby's tongue to the floor of his mouth is too short. It restricts the baby's tongue movement and can make it difficult for him to feed. Your paediatrician or midwife will check for tongue tie after your baby is born or during their first routine check but it is difficult to spot and can sometimes be missed. If your baby has mild tongue tie you may not experience any problems, however, in more serious cases it can affect breastfeeding for both you and your baby:

- Your baby may have difficulty latching on and is fretful when feeding.

- He may slide off your breast while feeding.

- He may not be gaining the amount of weight he should.

- You may suffer sore nipples, ulcers or bleeding.

If you are experiencing difficulties with breastfeeding, it is a good idea to rule out tongue tie as a cause so do ask your GP, midwife or health visitor to do a check. Although tongue tie is more commonly associated with breast-fed babies, occasionally a baby who is bottle-fed may experience problems when feeding. If your bottle-fed baby is fussy whilst feeding and displaying any of the following symptoms it is worthwhile having him checked out:

- Has problems latching onto the teat of the bottle properly and is fretful whilst feeding.

- Excessive milk leaking out the side of his mouth whilst feeding.

- He may not be gaining the amount of weight he should.

- Displays symptoms of colic.

- Excessive wind or hiccups during or after feeding.

- Clicking noise whilst feeding.

Tongue tie is treated with a simple operation in which the doctor will snip the base of the baby's tongue. If your baby is still very young he may not feel anything at all – the operation is generally performed without anaesthetic though in some cases a local anaesthetic will numb the area; he may even sleep through it. Older babies may need general aesthetic and the procedure is slightly more complex so ask your GP to explain it to you fully.

Common sleeping problems

Difficulties in settling

If your baby is difficult to settle at nap times, it is essential that you pay particular attention to the time you begin settling him and how long you spend trying to do this. With the majority of babies, the main reason they are hard to settle is overtiredness or overstimulation. Once you are confident that you have your baby's feeding and sleeping on track, I would strongly advise you to help your baby learn how to settle himself to sleep. Although it will be very difficult to listen to him cry, he will very quickly learn how to go to sleep by himself. He should never be left for more than 5–10 minutes before being checked. From my experience in helping thousands of parents with babies who have had serious sleeping problems, once a baby learns how to settle himself, he becomes happier and more relaxed. Once proper daytime sleep is established, night-time sleep will also improve. The following guidelines should help your baby learn how to settle himself:

- A baby who is allowed to fall asleep on the breast or bottle and is then put in the cot will be more likely to have disruptive nap times. When he comes into a light sleep 30–45 minutes after falling asleep, he will be less likely to settle himself back to sleep without your help. During the first few weeks, if your baby falls asleep while feeding, put him on the changing mat and rearrange his nappy. This should rouse him enough to go down in the cot semi-awake.

- Overtiredness is a major cause of babies not settling and not sleeping well during the day. Very young babies who are allowed to stay awake for longer than two hours at a time may get so overtired that they go on to fight sleep for a further two hours. The majority of babies, as they get older, will manage to stay awake slightly longer, sometimes up to two and a half hours at a time. A close eye should be kept on all babies after they have been awake for one and a half hours so that you do not miss the cue for sleep.

- Overhandling prior to sleep time is another major problem with young babies. Everyone wants just one little cuddle. Unfortunately, several little cuddles add up and can leave the baby fretful, overtired and difficult to settle. Your baby is not a toy. Do not feel guilty about restricting the handling in the early weeks, especially prior to sleep time.

- Overstimulation before sleep time is another major cause of babies not settling well. Babies under six months should be allowed a quiet wind-down time of 20 minutes before being put down to sleep. With babies over six months, avoid games and activities that cause them to get overexcited. With all babies, regardless of age, avoid excessive talking at put-down time. Talk quietly and calmly using the same simple phrases like 'night night' or 'its sleepy time now' along with a little shushing will help younger babies keep calm and settle more quickly, than getting into complicated conversation.

- The wrong sleep association can also cause long-term sleep problems. After a few weeks as your baby gets older it is essential that he goes down in his cot awake and learns to settle himself. For a baby who has already learned the wrong sleep associations, this problem can rarely be solved without some amount of crying. Fortunately, the majority of babies, if they are allowed, will learn to settle themselves within a few days.

Breast-fed baby not settling in the evening

By four weeks of age, some breast-fed babies start to become difficult to settle. They may go down sleepy and seem ready for sleep, but within 10 minutes have woken again.

- In my experience it is most likely that a breast-fed baby of this age is hungry. By offering him the breast again as soon as it becomes apparent to you that he is not going to settle, you should help prevent him becoming so distressed. Rather than trying to settle him by rocking him or offering him a dummy, offer him the breast that you fed him on at his last feed. Sometimes swapping the baby back and forth from both breasts at this time of day will encourage him to drink more.

- Babies of this age can also get very sleepy early evening, and keep falling asleep on the breast, but that does not mean that they are full. You may have to pick him up two or three times during the settling period and each time he should be offered the breast. If he then settles for the evening you will know that hunger is the main cause of the problem. If he is very sleepy at this time I would suggest that you offer most of the feed in a brightly lit room, before diming the lights for the last ten minutes of the feed.

- If he still doesn't settle despite being offered the breast several times, it could be that your milk supply is low at this time of the day. In that case it would be worth offering a bottle of expressed milk after his bath to see if that helps him settle any better (see page 176 for when to express for this feed).

- If despite increasing the milk your baby continues to be unsettled in the evening you should consider bringing his bedtime forward so that he is actually in bed slightly earlier. Next to hunger, overtiredness is one of the main causes of babies not settling in the evening. An earlier bedtime should ensure that he is not going down overtired, and along with more milk should help him fall into a relaxed sleep more easily.

- If your baby still continues to be unsettled in the evening, I would suggest that you follow the Assisting to sleep method (see below), as this will get your baby's body clock used to sleeping at the same time every night. Some parents are concerned that using this method will get their baby used to being held. However, getting their baby's body clock used to sleeping at the same time will, in the long term, make it easier to eventually settle him in his bed, instead of continuing to allow him to get into the habit of being awake on and off for three or four hours. After several nights of following the Assisting to sleep method, and when your baby is sleeping well between 7pm and 10pm, you should then find it easier to settle him in his bed.

Assisting to sleep method

All babies differ in how much sleep they need. During the first month some will feed, stay awake for a short period, then settle easily and sleep well until the next feed. However, if a baby gets into a pattern of sleeping well during the day and then not settling or sleeping well in the evening or at night, or is erratic with daytime naps, there are usually several reasons. Once you have ruled out genuine hunger as a cause, and are ensuring that your baby is well fed, I would advise that you try a solution that I call the 'assisting to sleep method'. The aim of this method is to get your baby used to sleeping at regular times during naps and in the evening, which will help him to sleep through the night as soon as he is physically able. After genuine hunger and the wrong sleep associations, I find that too much daytime sleep is the most common reason why a baby does not settle in the evening, or wakes frequently during the night. When this happens a vicious circle soon emerges where the baby needs to sleep more during the day because they are not sleeping well at night. In my experience, the only way to reverse this with a small baby is to assist the baby to sleep. Once their sleep improves in the night, a baby becomes much easier to keep awake during the day, which in turn has a knock-on effect on them sleeping better in the evening and at night. The aim of the assisting to sleep method is to get your baby used to sleeping at regular times during naps and in the evening. Once your baby is used to sleeping at the same times for several days, you should find that you can settle him in his bed with the minimum of fuss.

For this method to work it is important that it is done consistently and by only one parent. During stage one of the method, and for at least three days, do not attempt to put your baby in his bed at nap times or early evening. Instead, one parent should stay in a quiet room with him and cuddle him throughout the whole of the sleep-time.

Try to ensure that he is held in the crook of your arm, rather than lying across your chest. If he is older than two months and is no longer swaddled, it may help to use your right hand to hold both his hands across his chest; in this way, he will not wave his arms around and risk getting upset. It is important that the same person is with him during the allocated sleep time, and that you do not hand him back and forth, or walk from room to room. Once he is sleeping soundly for three days in a row at the recommended times, you should then progress onto the second stage and try to settle him in his bed. It is important to sit right next to his bed, so you can hold his hands across his chest and comfort him. On the fourth night, hold both his hands until he is asleep, and on the fifth night hold only one of his hands across his chest until he is asleep. By the sixth night you should find that you can put him down sleepy but awake in his bed, checking him every two or three minutes until he falls asleep. Do not try to settle him in his bed unless he has been sleeping soundly in your arms for at least three nights. Some babies may take longer than three days to sleep consistently at the recommended times.

When he reaches stage two, where he is settling within 10 minutes for several nights, you should try leaving him to self-settle using the crying down method described on page 352. It will help your baby get used to being happy in his bed if you put him in it for short spells during the day, when he is fully awake, with a small book or toy to look at. For the lunchtime nap, if you prefer, you can take your baby out for a nap in his pram or buggy. The important thing is to try to be consistent; the lunchtime nap should be in the buggy or in the home, but do not switch from one to the other midway through the nap.

Early-morning waking

All babies and young children come into a light sleep between 5–6am. Some will settle back to sleep for a further hour or so but many do not. I believe there are two things that determine whether a baby will become an earlier riser. One is the darkness of the room in which he sleeps. It would be an understatement to say I was obsessed with how dark the room should be, but I am totally convinced that it is the reason the majority of my babies quickly resettle themselves to sleep when they come into a light sleep at 5–6am. Once the door is shut and the curtains drawn, it should be so dark that not even the faintest trace of toys or books can be seen. A glimpse of these things will be enough to fully waken a baby from a drowsy state and make him want to start the day. How parents deal with early wakings during the first three months will also determine whether their baby will become a child who is an early riser. During the first few weeks, a baby who is waking and feeding at 2–2.30am may wake around 5–6am and genuinely need to feed. However, it is essential to treat this feed like a night-time feed. It should be done as quickly and quietly as possible with the use of only a small night-light and without talking or eye contact. The baby should then be settled back to sleep until 7–7.30am. If possible, avoid changing the nappy as this usually wakes the baby too much.

Once the baby is sleeping and feeding nearer 4am, waking at 6am is not usually related to hunger. This is the one and only time I would advise parents to help their baby return to sleep. At this stage the most important thing is to get him back to sleep quickly, even if it means cuddling him and offering him a dummy until 7am. Listed below are guidelines that will help your baby not to become an early riser:

- Avoid using a night-light or leaving the door open once you have put him down to sleep. Research shows that chemicals in the brain work differently in the dark, preparing it for sleep. Even the smallest chink of light can be enough to awaken the baby fully when he enters his light sleep.

- Kicking off the bedcovers can also cause babies under six months to wake early. In my experience, all babies under this age sleep better if tucked in securely. The sheet needs to be placed lengthways across the width of the cot to ensure that a minimum of 15cm (6in) is tucked in at the far side and a minimum of 10cm (4in) at the near side. I would also advise rolling up two small hand towels and pushing them down between the spars and the mattress on bothside.

- Babies who work their way up the cot and get out of the covers will benefit from being put in a very lightweight, 100 per cent cotton sleeping bag and tucked in with a sheet as described above. Depending on the weather, blankets may not be necessary.

- Once a baby starts to move around the cot and is capable of rolling both ways, I would advise that you remove the sheets and blankets and use only the sleeping bag. This will allow your baby to move around unrestricted, without the worry that he might get cold in the middle of the night. It is important to choose a sleeping bag that is suitable for the time of year.

- Do not drop the late feed until your baby is well established on solids. If he goes through a growth spurt before he starts solids, he can be offered extra milk at this time. This reduces the chances of waking early due to hunger, which can occur if the late feed is dropped too soon.

- If your baby is not fully established on solids, but is refusing a late feed, you may have to offer him a feed at 5–6am until solids are more established. Not many babies are capable of sleeping nearly twelve hours unless solids are fully established. Do not be tempted to try and push your baby through to 7am without a feed, as having a baby awake on and off at this time, is one of the main causes of early morning waking.

- A baby who is over six months and has dropped the late feed should be encouraged to stay awake until 7pm. If he is falling into a deep sleep before this time, he will be much more likely to wake before 7am.

Excessive night waking

Until the mother's milk comes in, a newborn baby may wake and need to be fed several times a night. By the end of the first week, a baby who weighs over 3.2kg (7lb) should manage to sleep for a longer stretch from the 10–11pm feed, provided his feeding needs are being fully met during the day. Smaller babies may still need to feed three-hourly around the clock. In my experience, all babies who are healthy and well fed will, between four and six weeks of age, manage to sleep for one longer spell of 4–6 hours. By following my routines this longer spell should happen in the night. The main aim of my routines is to help parents structure their baby's feeding and sleeping needs during the day so as to avoid excessive night waking and feeding.

How long a baby will continue to wake for a feed in the night depends very much on the individual baby. Some babies between six and eight weeks sleep through after the late feed, others between 10 and 12 weeks. Some may even take longer. All babies will sleep through the night as soon as they are physically and mentally able, provided the daytime feeding and sleeping is being properly structured. Listed below are the main causes of excessive night-time waking in healthy babies under one year old:

- Sleeping too much during the day. Even very small babies need to be awake some of the time. The baby should be encouraged to stay awake for one to one and a half hours after daytime feeds. Between 6 and 8 weeks most babies are capable of staying awake for one and a half to two hours, provided they are sleeping well in between feeds at night. At this stage try to ensure that your baby is awake properly for the late feed, so that the next waking in the night he will settle quickly. In my experience very young babies who are not awake fully at the late feed, tend to wake up much in the night, and even if not hungry, at this young age they are difficult to settle back without feeding.

- If excessive night feeding is to be avoided, babies under six months need to have 6–7 feeds between 7am and 11pm.

- Not feeding enough at each feed. In the early days most babies need up to 25 minutes on the first breast and if they are needing more than one feed between 11pm and 6–7am, then it is worth trying offering them the second breast, at least at some of the day time feeds.

- Breast-fed babies will be more likely to wake several times a night if they do not get enough to drink at the late feed and may need a top-up after this feed.

- Babies under six weeks have a very strong Moro reflex (see page 101) and can wake themselves several times a night by the sudden startle and jerk. In addition to being securely tucked in with an appropriate weight of sheet and blanket, these babies will benefit from being swaddled in a lightweight stretch-cotton sheet. Refer to pages 6–7 for how to ensure your baby's bed is made up so that he cannot kick his covers off.

- Older babies often wake several times at night because they have kicked their covers off and are cold, or they may have got their legs caught between the spars of the cot. A sleeping bag will help them avoid becoming cold and will prevent them from getting their legs caught in the spars.

- Between two and three months a baby's sleep cycle changes and during the day time sleep they move into a light sleep usually around 30–40 minutes after falling asleep. This also occurs several times a night. For babies who have learned to self-settle themselves, this will not be a problem. However, for those babies who have learned the wrong sleep associations, such as being fed, rocked or given a dummy to get to sleep, it is very likely that they will need the same assistance to resettle when they moves into a light sleep during a nap or in the night.

- For babies over six months, sleeping in their own room with a night-light on are more likely to be woken several times a night.

- If the baby's milk feeds are reduced too quickly when solids are introduced, he could begin to wake in the night genuinely needing a milk feed especially if the last feed is too low.

Sleepy late feed

Sleepy late feeds with very young babies can cause excessive night waking or early morning waking. In the early days, establishing a full feed at the late feed will help enormously in getting your baby to sleep for his longer spell during the night. Earlier in the book I advise that this feed should be a quiet feed in the nursery, so that the baby does not become overstimulated and then refuse to settle well. However, if your baby is so sleepy that he is not taking enough milk to get him to go one longer stretch in the night, then I would suggest that you introduce a split feed at the late feed. The success of the split feed depends on the baby being awake slightly longer, and drinking more milk. Some of the babies that I cared for were so sleepy in the early days that I would have to start waking them at 9.40–9.45pm. I would begin by switching on the light low, pulling back the covers, taking the baby's legs out of his sleep suit and then leaving him in his cot. I would allow 10 minutes and, if he was not starting to stir, I would then turn the light a little brighter. Regardless of how asleep he was, I would take him out of the room by 10pm at the latest. I would either take him to my bedroom or the sitting room, where I would have the lights, and possibly the television, switched on to create a more stimulating environment. I would then lay him on his play mat for a further 5–10 minutes if he was still not properly awake before I offered him the first bottle of his split feed. I would ensure that I made the formula slightly warmer than normal, and would always prepare a fresh bottle for the second half of the split feed, which I would give at 11.15pm. I would keep the baby as awake as possible between 10–11pm. With some babies it would often take up to two weeks to establish this split feed; but once it was established it really did help them take a bigger feed and sleep longer in the night.

If you are breast-feeding, the same method can be used, only you offer one breast at 10pm, followed by the second breast at 11.15pm. Some babies may actually need to have both breasts at 10pm, and then be offered the second breast again at 11.15pm – or perhaps a top-up of expressed milk if you feel your milk supply is low at this time.

If your baby is under 12 weeks, very sleepy and not feeding well at the last feed, it really is worth persevering with trying to establish a split feed. For this to work at the late feed, you would also have to be doing a split feed at 5–6.15pm. If you drop the split feed at this time, your baby will probably be taking a much bigger feed after his bath, which would have the knock-on effect of reducing his appetite at the late feed. If you have tried all of the suggestions above and your baby is still not feeding well and waking early in the night, you may wish to try dropping a late split feed for several nights and see how long he goes naturally. Once your baby sleeps a longer spell for several nights in a row, you would then re-introduce a late split feed and hopefully the baby will continue to sleep this longer spell but at the right time of night. Once he has slept through the night when doing a split feed for at least a week, you can gradually start to reduce the time he is awake by five minutes every two to three nights until he is taking a full feed in one go.

The majority of babies will continue to need at least one feed in the twelve-hour night until weaning is well established at around seven months of age. Therefore, it really is worthwhile being consistent and persistent about establishing a 10pm feed.

Illness – the effect on sleep

The majority of my first-born babies manage to get through the first year without suffering the usual colds and coughs that seem to plague my second-and third-born babies. By the time most first babies I have cared for experience a cold, their sleep is so well established that wakings in the night are very rare. With second and third babies this is not the case as they usually catch their first cold at a much younger age from a sibling and disrupted nights are inevitable. A baby under three months of age will usually need help to get through the night when they have a cold or are ill. A young baby with a cold can get very distressed, especially when he is feeding.

When a baby is sick, a night feed may need to be reintroduced if they are feeding poorly during the day. When I have had to care for a sick baby of over six months who wakes several times at night I find it less disruptive if I sleep in the same room as the baby. It enables me to attend to him quickly and I am less likely to interrupt the sleep of elder siblings by to-ing and fro-ing along the corridor. Occasionally, I find that an older baby who has dropped night-time feeds will, once he has recovered, continue to wake up in the night looking for a feed or the same attention he received when he was unwell.

For the first few nights I would check him and offer him some cool boiled water, but once I was convinced he was totally recovered, I would leave him time to settle himself. In my experience, parents who are not prepared to do this usually end up with a baby who develops a long-term sleep problem. If your baby develops a cold or cough, regardless of how mild it appears, he should be seen by a doctor. All too often I hear from distressed parents of babies with serious chest infections, which could possibly have been avoided if they had been seen by a doctor earlier. Too many parents delay taking their baby to the doctor, worried that they will be classed as neurotic, but it is important that you discuss with your doctor any concerns you have about your baby's health, however small. If your baby is ill, it is essential that you follow your doctor's advice to the letter, especially on feeding.

The lunchtime nap

The lunchtime nap is a fundamental part of my CLB routines. Research shows that babies and young children benefit from a proper, structured nap in the middle of the day. As your baby grows and is more active, this nap will become his time to rest and recover from the morning's activities and will enable him to enjoy his afternoons with you and others.

However, I am well aware that in the early days a lunchtime nap can sometimes go wrong. I understand the feelings of frustration when a baby wakes 30–45 minutes into the nap and, despite still being tired, refuses to settle back to sleep. Assuming that the wrong sleep associations have not been established, there are several things you can do to try to improve the lunchtime nap. The first thing is to allow your baby a short time to settle himself back to sleep, provided you are confident that the waking is not due to genuine hunger. Normally, over a period of a week or so, if a baby is allowed 5–10 minutes of crying down, they will then start to settle themselves back to sleep. Obviously, if you find that after 10 minutes your baby is not crying down but is in fact crying up, then he should be attended to. With a baby who is crying up, I would offer half of the 2pm feed, treating it like a night feed, so that the baby does not become overstimulated by lots of talking or eye contact. I would then assume that the reason why the baby can't settle himself back to sleep is because his coming into a light sleep coincides with him starting to get hungry.

Hunger – younger babies

To eliminate the possibility of hunger causing a disturbed lunchtime nap, I would bring forward the morning feed for very young babies to 10–10.30am, and then offer a top-up just before they go down for their nap. This way you can be confident about allowing them a short crying down period, without worrying that they might be hungry.

If they continue to cry up and not settle back to sleep, it is worth looking at the amount of sleep your baby is having at the morning nap.

Morning nap – younger babies

If your baby is between one and six months, and having more than one hour of sleep in the morning, it could be that too much morning sleep is affecting his lunchtime nap. Depending on how much sleep your baby is having at the morning nap, I would try reducing it to between 45 minutes and 1 hour, maximum. Occasionally, with some babies over three months I have had to reduce the morning nap to only 30 minutes to ensure a two-hour nap at lunchtime. If you find that you cannot push your baby on to 9am for his morning nap, I would suggest that you do a split morning nap for a short time in order to reduce his overall morning sleep time. Allow him 20–30 minutes at the first part of the split nap, then a further 10–15 minutes at the second part of the split nap. By offering your baby a top-up before his lunchtime nap, reducing his morning nap to between 30–40 minutes and allowing him a short spell of crying down when he does wake after only 45 minutes, he should start to sleep for a longer spell again.

Hunger – older babies

With a baby who is weaned, you can try offering a top-up of milk just prior to his lunchtime nap. If you find that he is taking quite a large top-up, it would be worth looking at the amount of solids that you are giving, and ensure that you are getting the right balance of protein, carbohydrates and vegetables. By seven months, your baby should be eating three meals a day and solids should be well-established. Check *The Contented Little Baby Book of Weaning* for the recommended amounts and meal planners. If you have weaned at six months, you will need to move through the guide quickly to build up the right amounts of food. In my experience most babies aged 6–9 months need between six and eight tablespoons of solids at each meal. If your baby is getting less than this, then hunger could be the cause. If your baby is over nine months and is not having a good drink of water with his lunch, thirst can be a reason why he wakes up early from his nap, especially during hot weather. It is, therefore, worth offering him a drink of water just prior to his lunchtime nap.

Once the possibility of hunger is ruled out, if your baby continues to cry up instead of down, then you should look at the amount of sleep your baby is having in the morning.

Morning nap – older babies

With babies over six months, try to ensure that the morning nap is not before 9.15–9.30am. If you find your baby is sleeping longer than 45 minutes at this nap, this could be the reason for him not sleeping so long at lunchtime.

If your baby is between six and nine months, it is important to push the morning nap on until 9.30am and reduce the morning nap gradually, cutting it back by 10 minutes every three or four days until he is having only 20–25 minutes. If your baby is between nine and twelve months, try reducing it to 10–15 minutes, or cutting out the nap entirely. You may find that for a short time you will have to bring his lunch and nap forward slightly if he is getting tired and put him down earlier. The top-up before the nap and the reduction in the morning sleep should see an improvement in the length of time he sleeps at the lunchtime nap within one or two weeks. Refer to pages 240–245 on how reduce and eliminate the morning nap.

The lunchtime nap – further trouble-shooting

If you find that your baby will not resettle back to sleep at the lunchtime nap, despite trying all the suggestions above, you will have to adjust the routine for his afternoon sleep, so that he does not become overtired at bedtime. The age of your baby will dictate how much sleep you give him later in the day. A younger baby may need a 30-minute nap after the 2.30pm feed, and then a further short nap at around 4.30pm. This should stop him getting overtired and irritable and help you to get his routine back on track again by 5pm, so that he settles well at 7pm. Sometimes a baby doesn't sleep at 2.30pm, especially if over nine months old, but will then fall asleep later, between 3–4pm, and then wake after 30–45 minutes. If this happens, you may find that you have to bring bedtime forward slightly. The important thing to remember when adjusting the routines to make up for a shorter lunchtime nap is to try to follow the recommendations for the maximum amount of daily sleep for your baby's age. Also, try to make sure that your baby is up and awake by 5pm if you want him to go down well at 7pm.

Checklist

- Rule out hunger as the possible cause of waking by offering a top-up milk feed just prior to the nap. If an older baby who is weaned is drinking more than a couple of ounces (60ml), it is possible he needs his solids to be increased. Some breast-fed babies, despite eating a good amount of solids, may need a top-up breast feed until past nine months of age.

- With an older baby, check he is not thirsty by offering him a drink of cool boiled water just before he goes down for his lunchtime nap.

- Correct any sleep associations, such as falling asleep on the breast or the bottle, and ensure he goes down, well-fed, in his bed. It might take some time to get your baby into good habits, so you will need to be patient.

- Eliminate all other reasons for waking, such as excessive noise or young babies not being tucked in properly. (Remember that the Moro reflex – see page 101 – can be very strong in babies under six months, so tucking them in securely is very important if they are not to wake themselves up.)

- Always allow your baby to wake up naturally and, after the first few weeks, provided he is not screaming for food, allow him a short awake spell in his bed before you pick him up; in this way, he will not associate waking with being picked up immediately.

When you have checked everything on the list above, and given any changes enough time to work, if the lunchtime nap still continues to be a problem (and you feel your baby has got into the habit of waking when he comes into a light sleep) it may be worth trying the assisting to sleep method, mentioned on page 337. This method can help babies to sleep at regular times. I would also suggest checking out *The Complete Sleep Guide for Contented Babies and Toddlers*, which has extensive advice and lots of case studies on sleeping problems.

Crying down at the lunchtime nap

In my books I say that 'crying down' can be used from a very young age with babies who fight sleep or are overtired. It is very important to understand the difference between crying down and sleep training so that your baby is not caused any distress and the problem you are struggling with is not made worse. Below is a brief summary of the method:

Crying down is appropriate when a baby who is well-fed, tired and ready to sleep fights sleep when put in the cot. They will usually cry on and off for 5–10 minutes before drifting off to sleep – although some very overtired babies may cry on and off for up to 20 minutes. Once asleep, these babies will then sleep for the full nap time, or at night until the next feed is due. If your baby wakes after 30–45 minutes and then settles back within 10–20 minutes of fussing for a further 30–45 minutes, this could be classed as crying down. But if your baby wakes up after 30–45 minutes, does not settle back to sleep and is left to cry for longer than the suggested time, then this is *not* crying down. I do not recommend that babies be left to cry for lengthy periods, as this not only causes distress, but creates a habit of them crying the minute they wake up or come into a light sleep. It is much better to get the baby up and allow him either one or two short naps later in the afternoon, depending on his age. In my experience, as long as parents establish the right sleep associations and learn how to adjust the afternoon nap so that their baby does not become overtired, their baby will eventually start to sleep longer at the lunchtime nap.

Sleep associations

During the early months many babies are happy to doze on and off in a baby seat or Moses basket, which can be convenient as it allows parents more flexibility. Unfortunately, once the baby becomes bigger and more active, he is unlikely to continue to sleep well or for long enough in the baby seat. If this habit is established it can be very difficult to get him to sleep in his cot during the day. The sleep in the baby seat is unlikely to be satisfying and, as he gets older, he will most likely spend the time catnapping and become tired and irritable later on. The knock-on effect of this is that he might not feed well at teatime or fall asleep before he's had all of his bedtime milk. Night wakings due to hunger can then result, leaving all of you tired the next day and so the problem continues to get worse.

If sleep associations and an erratic sleeping pattern have taken root, you will need to focus on getting him to sleep during this nap period. This is known as Assisting the baby to sleep method (see page 337). Take him out in the buggy or the car, and let him have the two hours he needs. I usually found that if I did this for a week or even 10 days, the baby's sleep cycle would adapt to it and it was easier then to put him down in his cot with just a little bit of 'crying down'. For further information on sleep associations and how to deal with them, please check out contentedbaby.com.

Teething and night waking

In my experience, babies who enjoy a routine from a very early age and have established healthy sleeping habits are rarely bothered by teething. Out of the hundreds of babies I have helped care for, only a handful have been bothered by teething in the night. In these cases it is usually when the molars come through and then only for a few nights. I have found that babies who wake in the night due to teething are more likely to have suffered from colic and have developed poor sleeping habits.

If your baby is teething and waking in the night but quickly settles back to sleep when given a cuddle or a dummy, teething is probably not the real cause of his waking. A baby who is genuinely bothered by teething pain would be difficult to settle back to sleep. He would also show signs of discomfort during the day, not just at night. I would advise you to check the section on excessive night waking and early-morning waking to eliminate other reasons for your baby waking.

If you are convinced that your baby's night-time wakings are caused by severe teething pain, I suggest you seek advice from your doctor regarding the use of paracetamol and ibuprofen. While genuine teething pain may cause a few disruptive nights, it should never last for several weeks. If your baby seems out of sorts, develops a fever and suffers from loss of appetite or diarrhoea, he should be seen by a doctor. Do not assume that these symptoms are just a sign of teething. Very often I have found that what parents thought was teething turned out to be an ear or throat infection.

Sleep regression

Having worked with babies for over thirty years, I found that once they were in a good routine and sleeping through the night, apart from illness, they would continue to sleep well at night. Out of the hundreds of babies I helped care for personally, and the thousands of babies I have advised upon through my consultancy, I have never had parents coming back to me saying their baby's sleep has regressed – until recently that is. I now find that am getting an increasing number of emails from parents asking for advice on how to deal with their baby's sleep regression. On researching further into what "sleep regression" is, it appears that some people believe that at certain ages babies go through a developmental stage that can affect their sleep, resulting in them waking up in the night again. My own personal view is that sleep only regresses if parents are not one step ahead of their baby's ever-changing feeding and sleeping needs. If there were such a thing as genuine "sleep regression" due to developmental changes, then I am convinced that from the thousands of parents that I have advised, at least some of them would have come back to me and said that their baby's sleep keeps back-tracking. Indeed it has been the complete opposite: I hear on a regular basis from parents I advised, often many years ago, how well their child has continued to sleep. If your baby has experienced what you believe to be sleep regression, I would urge you to check the nine different routines found in this book. The reason I offer these nine different routines is because I believe that a baby's needs keep changing during the first year, and those parents who are one step ahead of their baby's needs will use the routines to ensure that their baby's feeding and sleeping needs are adapted and gradually changed before things go wrong.

Golden rules

Finally, here are some essential tips to avoid potential problems in the first year:

- In the early days I advise that babies can stay awake for up to two hours. This does not mean that they should be awake for two hours. If your baby settles to sleep well in the evening and after night feeds, but can only stay awake for an hour or so at a time during the day, he is obviously a baby who needs more sleep. However, if your baby is not settling well in the evening, or after feeds in the middle of the night, and you have ruled out the possibility of hunger, then it would be worth gradually lengthening your baby's awake time by a couple of minutes every few days until he can stay awake happily for longer and sleep better in the night.

- I recommend that babies *should* be allowed up to 25 minutes on the first breast, not that they *must* have 25 minutes on the breast. Some babies are very efficient feeders and can take a full feed in much less time. If your baby is gaining weight and settling to sleep well for daytime naps and at night, then you do not need to worry how long he is on the breast for. However, if your baby is unhappy between feeds and not settling well for naps, it's possible that he is not taking a full feed. Try offering him the breast just prior to naps. If he then settles well you can be fairly sure that hunger is the cause of him not settling. To remedy this I would advise seeking help from a professional breast-feeding counsellor to ensure that you are latching your baby onto the breast properly. Once you are confident about this, you should keep checking that he is actually swallowing and not just sucking when he is feeding. Very small babies who spend lots of time sucking instead of feeding can quickly become tired and pull off the breast before they have taken a full feed.

- In the early days, if your baby is crying you should always assume it is hunger and feed him. Remember, when I talk about three-hourly feeding the three hours are calculated from the beginning of one feed, to the beginning of the next feed. This means there is only a two-hour gap between feeds. I also say that, if a baby is genuinely hungry before the recommended feed times, they should always be fed. However, if your baby is looking for a feed long before the recommended time for his age, you should also try to work out why. The cause with breast-fed babies is usually a low milk supply or the baby not taking enough at feeds. If your baby is formula-fed and not managing to go three hours between feeds, you should discuss whether he is taking enough at each feed with your health visitor.

- Do not move on to the next routine until your baby shows signs that he is ready to stay awake longer and go longer between feeds. Depending on your baby's individual needs, you may find that your baby is sometimes between two routines. This may result in following sleeping times from one routine and feeding times from the next, or vice versa, but this is fine.

- Remember, the aim of the routines is to establish healthy long-term sleeping and feeding habits. A baby will sleep through the night as soon as he is physically and mentally able. You should not try to push your baby through the night by restricting or reducing night feeds too quickly.

- To avoid early-morning waking, ensure that in the early days when your baby wakes in the night you give him a big enough feed to get him through to nearer 7am. Also, once he is sleeping to 5–6am you should not leave him for lengthy periods to see if he will settle back to sleep. A baby who gets into the habit of being awake for any length of time between 5–7am is much more likely to develop a long-term early-morning waking problem than a baby who is fed quickly and settled back to sleep.

- It is also important that you do not reduce the time your baby is awake at the late feed until he is sleeping regularly to nearer 7am. If he reaches two months and is not sleeping until nearer 7am, it is worth splitting the late feed and having him awake longer at that time. In my experience, the split feed nearly always helped very young babies sleep longer in the night; with older babies who were waking up at 5am, it helped them sleep nearer to 7am. Refer to page 173 for details of how to implement the split feed, and allow at least a week to establish it. The key to the success of the split feed is ensuring that you wake the baby no later than 9.45pm and keep him fully awake for the recommended time.

- Babies over six months who have dropped the late feed and start to wake up between 5–6am but do not settle back to sleep within 10–15 minutes, should be offered a feed, even if the cause is not hunger. In my experience feeding the baby the minute they wake is the quickest way to avoid long-term early morning waking. At the age when solids are established, too much daytime sleep is usually the cause of early morning waking. Trying to reduce daytime sleep with a baby who is waking early is very difficult, hence the reason for offering a feed as, unlike offering a dummy or cuddles, it allows the baby to settle himself back to sleep. Then, as the baby sleeps better between 5–7am, gradually push the 9am nap on to 9.30am and reduce it to 30 minutes. This will then enable you to push the lunchtime nap on to 12.30pm and will eliminate any late afternoon nap. Once your baby's daytime sleep is reduced you will probably find that he will naturally start to sleep to nearer 7am and drop the early morning feed. However, if he has been sleeping through to nearer 7am for at least two weeks and you find that you are still feeding between him between 5–6am, you can start to reduce the amount of milk you give him. Once you reach a stage where he is settling back with the only the smallest feed, you can then drop the feed and allow him to settle himself back to sleep.

Appendix

The Lullaby Trust Advice to reduce the risk of cot death:

1. During the night and day for the first six months, place your baby to sleep on his back in a suitable bed with a flat and firm mattress in a room with you.

2. Babies do not need hot rooms; all-night heating is rarely necessary. Keep the room at a temperature between 16–20ºC (61–68ºF); 18ºC (65°F) is just right.

3. Adults find it difficult to judge the temperature of a room, so use a room thermometer in the rooms where your baby sleeps and plays. A simple room thermometer is available from The Lullaby Trust.

4. When you check your baby, if he is sweating or his tummy feels hot to the touch, take off some of the bedding.

5. Use lightweight blankets or a baby sleeping bag. If your baby feels too warm, reduce the number of layers or use a lower tog baby sleeping bag. In a warm summer, your baby may not need any bedclothes at all. Do not use a baby nest, a duvet, quilt or pillow for babies under 12 months.

6. Even in winter, babies who are unwell and feverish need fewer clothes and bedclothes.

7. Babies need to lose excess heat from their heads. Make sure his head cannot be covered by the bedclothes by sleeping

him 'feet to foot' (with his feet to the foot of the cot) so he doesn't wriggle down under the covers.

8. It is very important that babies do not have soft toys, muslins or comforters in their beds.

The Lullaby Trust Advice on car seats and young babies:

1. Avoid travelling in cars with pre-term and very young babies for long periods of time. Ideally, a second adult should travel in the back of the car with the baby or a mirror should be used so the driver can keep an eye on the baby at all times.

2. If a baby changes its position and slumps forward, then parents should immediately stop and take the baby out of the car seat.

For more information please visit: lullabytrust.org.uk and nhs.uk.

Useful Addresses

Baby equipment

The Great Little Trading Company
PO Box 336
Birkenhead CH25 9DN
Tel: 0844 848 6000
gltc.co.uk

Blackout lining and blinds

Easyblinds
Brook Farm
Sotherton
Beccles
Suffolk IP19 8NW
Tel: 01986 875099
easyblindsonline.co.uk

Bottles and cups

BabyBornFree Ltd
Building 3 – Chiswick Park
566 Chiswick High Road
London W4 5YA
Tel: 020 8732 4728
babybornfree.co.uk

Breast pumps

ardomedical.co.uk
ardobreastpumps.co.uk

Organisations

FSA (Food Standards Agency)
Aviation House
125 Kingsway
London WC2B 6NH
Tel: 020 7276 8000
food.gov.uk

La Leche League
PO Box 29
West Bridgford
Nottingham NG2 7NP
Tel: 0845 456 1855
Helpline: 0845 120 2918
laleche.org.uk

The Lullaby Trust (Advice and support on sudden infant death)
11 Belgrave Road
London SW1V 1RB
Tel: 020 7802 3200
lullabytrust.org.uk

NCT (National Childbirth Trust)
Alexandra House
Oldham Terrace
Acton

London W3 6NH
Tel: 0300 330 0770
nct.org.uk

TAMBA (Twins and Multiple Births Association)
2 The Willows
Gardner Road
Guildford
Surrey GU1 4PG
Tel: 01483 304442
tamba.org.uk

Further Reading

A Contented House with Twins by Gina Ford and Alice Beer (Vermilion 2006)

Feeding Made Easy by Gina Ford (Vermilion 2008)

From Crying Baby to Contented Baby by Gina Ford (Vermilion 2010)

Gina Ford's Top Tips for Contented Babies and Toddlers by Gina Ford (Vermilion 2006)

Healthy Sleep Habits, Happy Child by Marc Weissbluth (Vermilion 2005)

Potty Training in One Week by Gina Ford (Vermilion 2003)

Remotely Controlled by Aric Sigman (Vermilion 2005)

Silent Nights by Brian Symon (OUP Australia and New Zealand 2005)

Sleep: The Secret of Problem-free Nights by Beatrice Hollyer and Lucy Smith (Cassell 2002)

Solve Your Child's Sleep Problems by Richard Ferber (Dorling Kindersley 1985)

The Complete Sleep Guide for Contented Babies and Toddlers by Gina Ford (Vermilion 2006)

The Contented Baby with Toddler Book by Gina Ford (Vermilion 2009)

The Contented Baby's First Year by Gina Ford (Vermilion 2007)

The Contented Child's Food Bible by Gina Ford (Vermilion 2005)

The Contented Little Baby Book of Weaning by Gina Ford (Vermilion 2006)

The Contented Toddler Years by Gina Ford (Vermilion 2006)

The Gina Ford Baby and Toddler Cook Book by Gina Ford (Vermilion 2005)

The Great Ormond Street New Baby and Child Care Book (Vermilion 2004)

The New Baby and Toddler Sleep Programme by Professor John Pearce with Jane Biddler (Vermilion 1999)

What to Expect When You're Breast-feeding ... And What If You Can't? by Clare Byam-Cook (Vermilion 2006)

Your Child's Symptoms Explained by David Haslam (Vermilion 1997)

contentedbaby.com

Would you like to learn more about the Contented Baby routines and Gina Ford's books? Why not visit Gina's official website at contentedbaby.com. As a member you'll find there are a huge range of benefits as well as a wealth of information and advice.

The membership benefits of joining the only official Gina Ford website include:

- Access to our regularly updated database of over 2,000 FAQs on feeding, sleeping and development answered by Gina and other childcare experts.

- More than 40 case studies on feeding, sleeping and development.

- An archive of over 300 features from recognized writers, nutritionists, psychologists and counsellors on parenting and lifestyle issues.

- Regular online magazine with a personal message from Gina and access to Gina's problem page.

- *Gina responds* – a page where Gina responds to the most common concerns posted by members.

- Popular recipes and menu planners for babies and toddlers.

INDEX

addresses, useful 361–3
adjusting the routines *see*
    Contented Little Baby
    (CLB) routines
assisting to sleep method 166, 294,
    337–9, 352

baby equipment 10–17, 361 *see*
    also equipment, baby
bath, baby 13–14
beaker, introducing a 271
bedding, cot 5–8
bedtime routine 97–100
birth, preparation for the 1–31
Bisphenol A (BPA) 20
boredom 298
bottle-feeding:
    CLB routines and *see* Contented
        Little Baby (CLB) routines
    equipment needed for 21–3
        bottle brush 22
        feeding bottles 20–1
        kettle 23
        steriliser 22–3
        teat brush 22
        teats 21
        washing-up bowl 22
    establishing 76–81
        giving the feed 79–81
        hygiene and sterilisation 77–8
    formula: overfeeding 83
    successful 81–2
    weaning your baby from the
        breast to the bottle 71–3
breakfast, introducing 269–70,
    276–7, 280

breast pads 18
breast-feeding/breast-fed babies:
    breast-fed baby not settling in
        the evening 336–7
    chart for the first year 130–1
    CLB routines and *see* Contented
        Little Baby (CLB) routines
    diluting feeds 84–5
    equipment needed for 18–21
        breast pads 18
        feeding bottles 20–1
        freezer bags 19–20
        nipple cream and sprays 19
        nursing bra 18
        nursing pillow 18
    expressing and 64–7
    feeding problems, common
        311–34 *see also* feeding
        problems, common
    first year 54–90
    formula: overfeeding 83
    milk composition 58–60
    milk let-down reflex 57–8
    milk oversupply 67–9
    milk production 57–60
    milk supply, plan for increased
        314–19
    my methods for successful 61–4,
        62
    questions answered, your 85–90
    refusal of milk 327–8
    returning to work and 69–71
    sleeping problems and 334, 336–
        7, 343, 345, 351, 356, 357
    structuring the milk feeds during
        the first year 114–16

breast-feeding/breast-fed babies:
(*continued*)
weaning your baby and 71–3,
257, 258, 259, 260, 269,
270, 272, 273, 274, 278,
279, 280, 284, 286, 292
weaning your baby from the
breast to the bottle 71–3
why breast-feeding goes wrong
55–7
see also bottle-feeding
burping 291–3
Byam-Cook, Clare: *What to
Expect When You're
Breast-Feeding ... And
What If You Can't?* 57, 61

car seat 12–13, 16, 162, 305, 360
cardigans 25
carpeting 9
chairs 8–9, 16–17
changing mat 14
changing station 8
CLB routines *see* Contented Little
Baby (CLB) routines
clothes for the newborn 23–8
cardigans 25
day outfits 25
hats 26
jacket 28
mittens 26
nightwear 25
snowsuit 28
socks 26
swaddling blanket 26–8
vests 24–5
colic 21, 59, 62, 88, 293–4, 298,
302–3, 333, 354
contentedbaby.com xvi, xvii, 28,
69, 130, 163, 305, 317, 366
Contented Little Baby (CLB)
routines xvi, xvii, 32
adjusting the routines 146–61
birth to six months 146–7

for daytime outings 150–7
for evenings out 154–7
for holidays 157–61
for nursery 148–50
six months onwards 147
cuddling and 113
daytime sleep during the first
year, structuring 131–46
establishing xvi, 108–63
feeding and 108–10
feeding, understanding the
routines for 116–31
6–7am feed 116–19
10–11am feed 119–21
2.30pm feed 121–2
6–7pm feed 122–4
late feed 124–7
milk feeding chart for the first
year 130–1
night feeds 127–30
late-afternoon nap 144–6
lunchtime nap 141–4
milk feeds during the first year,
structuring the 114–16
months three to four 221–30
see also months three to
four
months four to six 231–9 *see
also* months four to six
months six to nine 240–8 *see
also* six to nine
months nine to twelve 249–56
see also nine to twelve
nap times, importance of 132–3
playing and 112–13
settling your baby, important
recommendations 162–3
sleep required during the first
year, guide to 162
sleeping and 110–12
sleeping routine, understanding
the 133–41
weeks one to two 164–75 *see
also* weeks one to two

weeks two to four 176–87 *see also* weeks two to four
weeks four to six 188–99 *see also* weeks four to six
weeks six to eight 200–11 *see also* weeks six to eight
weeks eight to twelve 212–20 *see also* weeks eight to twelve
why follow a routine? 32–53
   benefits for you 35–6
   benefits for your baby 34–5
   demand feeding 38–40
   other approaches 36–53
   questions answered, your 41–53
   strict four-hourly feeding routine 36–8
   why the CLB routines are different 33–4
   why they are different? 33–4
cot, the 1, 2, 4–8
   bedding 5–8
   making up the 6–8
cot death, risk of 5, 27, 162–3, 195–6, 299, 301, 359–60
crying 45–6, 294–8
   crying down at the lunchtime nap 352–3
cuddling 44–5, 113
curtains 9

daily requirements, solid food 272–4, 278–9, 282–4
day outfits 25
daytime outings, adjusting the routine for 150–7
   evening routine at a friend's house 152
   evenings out, adjusting the routine for 154–7
   fresh air and exercise 153
   lunch, managing sleeping and naps when going out to 151–2

next day after social event 153
   socialising, guidelines for successful 155–7
daytime sleep, structuring during the first year 131–46 *see also* sleep
decoration, nursery 3–4
defrosting tips 264
demand feeding 20, 38–40, 41–2, 43, 45, 54, 109, 293, 298, 314
   sleep and 94–5
Department of Health (DoH) 3, 162, 257
difficult feeder 311–12
diluting feeds 84–5
dummies 299–301

early-morning waking 100–3, 339–41, 354, 357
equipment, baby 10–17
   baby bath 13–14
   baby monitor, choosing 14–15
   car seat 12–13
   chair, baby 16–17
   changing mat 14
   Moses basket or small crib 10
   playpen 17
   pram 11–12
   sling, baby 15–16
evenings out, adjusting the routine for 154–7
excessive night feeding 108, 319–24, 343
excessive night waking 342–6, 354
expressing 64–7
   CLB routines and *see* Contented Little Baby (CLB) routines
   electric expressing machine 19

feeding:
   bottle-feeding *see* bottle-feeding
   breast-feeding *see* breast-feeding
   CLB routines and *see* Contented Little Baby (CLB) routines

feeding: (*continued*)
common feeding problems
311–34
demand feeding 20, 38–40, 41,
43, 45, 54, 94–5, 109, 293,
298, 314
four-hourly feeding routine,
strict 36–8
milk feeding in the first year 54–90
solid food, introducing 257–90
first year:
guide to sleep required during
the 162
milk feeding chart for the 130–1
milk feeding in the 54–90
problem-solving 291–358
structuring daytime sleep during
the 131–46
structuring the milk feeds
during the 114–16
see also Contented Little Baby
(CLB) routines
foods:
to be avoided 88, 260–2
to introduce 268–9, 275–6
preparing and cooking food for
your baby 262–4
see also feeding
formula: overfeeding 83
four-hourly feeding routine, strict
36–8
freezer:
bags 19–20
packing food for the 263
fresh air and exercise 153
friend's house, evening routine at
a 152
fussy feeder 329–32

general problems 291–310
Gina Ford Personal Telephone
Consultancy xvii
giving the feed 79–81
golden rules 355–8

hats 26
Herman, Professor John 132–3
hiccups 301–2
holidays, adjusting the routine for
157–61
helping your baby adjust to
a different time change
158–61
travelling from London to
Mauritius 160–1
hunger 296–7, 348, 349
hygiene and sterilisation 77–8

illness, sleep and 346–7
ironing 31

jacket 28

kettle 23

late-afternoon nap 133, 144–6
eight to twelve weeks 145–6
first month 145
four to eight weeks 145
three months onwards 146
late feed, the 124–7
laundry, your baby's 29–31
corduroy and dark clothes 31
dark colours: 30°C or
handwash 30
ironing 31
light colours: 40°C 30
tumble dryer, use of 30
whites: 60–90°C 29
wollens or delicates: handwash
30
lighting 10
London to Mauritius, travelling
from 160–1
low milk supply 313–14
Lullaby Trust 3, 11, 13, 27, 162,
163, 299, 301, 362
Advice on Car Seats and Young
babies 360

Advice to Reduce the Risk of
Cot Death 359–60
lunch 277, 280–1
managing sleeping and naps
when going out to 151–2
lunchtime nap 141–4, 208–9,
347–53
checklist 351
crying down at the 352–3
eight to twelve weeks 143
first month 141–2
four to eight weeks 142–3, 208–9
hunger and 348, 349
morning nap and 348–9, 350
nine to twelve months 144
problem solving 347–53
six months onwards 144
three to six months 143

milk feeding in the first year 54–90
bottle-feeding *see* bottle-feeding
breast-feeding *see* breast-feeding
chart for the first year 130–1
diluting feeds 84–5
expressing 64–7
formula: overfeeding 83
in the first year 54–90
milk composition 58–60
milk oversupply 67–9
milk production 57–60
plan for increased milk supply
314–19
refusal of milk 327–8
water to babies under six
months, giving 83–4
weaning your baby from the
breast to the bottle 71–3
your questions answered 85–90
mittens 26
monitor, choosing baby 14–15
months three to four 221–30
changes to be made during the
three-to four-month routine
225–30

feeding 227–30
sleeping 225–7
routine – three to four months
221–30
7am 221
8am 222
9am 222
9.45am 222
10am 222
11am 222
11.50am 222
12 noon–2/2.15pm 223
2/2.15pm 223
4/4.15pm 223–4
5pm 224
5.45pm 224
6pm 224
6.15pm 224
7pm 225
8pm 225
9.30pm 225
10/10.30pm 225
months four to six 231–9
changes to be made during the
four-to six-month routine
235–9
feeding 237–9
sleeping 235–7
routine – four to six months
231–9
7am 231
8am 231–2
9/9.15am 232
9.45am 232
10am 232
11am 232
11.50am 232
12/12.15pm 233
2/2.15pm 233
4.15pm 233
5pm 233–4
5.30pm 234
5.45pm 234
6/6.15pm 234

months four to six (*continued*)
  7pm 235
  9.30pm 235
  10pm 235
months six to nine 240–8
  changes to be made during the
    six-to nine-month routine
    244–8
  feeding 245–8
  sleeping 244–5
  routine – six to nine months
    240–3
  7am 241
  8am 241
  9.15/9.30am 241
  9.55am 241
  11.30am 242
  12.20pm 242
  12.30pm–2.30pm 242
  2.30pm 242–3
  4.15pm 243
  5pm 243
  6pm 243
  6.30pm 243
  7pm 243
months nine to twelve 249–56
  changes to be made during
    the nine-to twelve-month
    routine 253–6
  cutting out the morning nap
    254–5
  feeding 255–6
  sleeping 253–4
  routine – nine to twelve months
    249–53
  7am 249
  8am 250
  9.30am 250
  9.55am 250
  11.45am/12 noon 250
  12.20pm 250–1
  2.30pm 251
  4.15pm 251
  5pm 252

6.15/6.30pm 252
6.30pm 252
7pm 253
Moses basket or small crib 2, 4, 8,
  10–11, 13, 162, 353

naps:
  crying down at the lunchtime
    nap 352–3
  importance of 132–3
  late-afternoon nap 133, 144–6
  lunchtime nap 141–4, 208–9,
    347–53
  managing sleeping and naps when
    going out to lunch 151–2
  splitting 137
night feeds, the 127–30
nightwear 25
nipple cream and sprays 19
nursery 1, 2, 3–4
  carpeting 9
  chair 8–9
  changing station 8
  cot, the 4–8
  curtains 9
  decoration 4–5
  lighting 10
  wardrobe 8
nursery school, adjusting the
    routine for 148–50
  feeding 149–50
  sleeping 148–9
nursing bra 18

older babies 15, 157, 313, 334,
  343, 358
  hunger 349
  morning nap 350
  starting the routine with 166
overtiredness 40, 52, 132, 139, 173,
  294, 297–8, 334, 335, 337

pillow, nursing 18
playing 112–13

playpen 17
posseting 302–3
pram 11–12
premature babies, starting the
    routine with 165–6
preparing and cooking food for
    your baby 262–4
problem-solving in the first year
    291–358
  common feeding problems
    311–34
    difficult feeder 311–12
    excessive night feeding 319–24
    fussy feeder 329–32
    low milk supply 313–14
    plan for increased milk supply
      314–19
    refusal of milk 327–8
    rcfusal of solids 328–9
    sleepy feeder 324–6
    tongue tie 332–4
  common sleeping problems
    334–58
    assisting to sleep method
      337–9
    breast-fed baby not settling in
      the evening 336–7
    difficulties in settling 334–5
    early-morning waking 339–41
    excessive night waking 342–6
    golden rules 355–8
    illness, sleep and 346–7
    lunchtime nap 347–53
    sleep associations 353
    sleep regression 354–5
    teething and night waking
      353–4
  general problems 291–310
    burping 291–3
    colic 293–4
    crying 294–8
    dummies 299–301
    hiccups 301–2
    posseting 302

reflux 302–5
  separation anxiety 306–9
  stranger anxiety 309–10
protein at lunchtime, introducing
    270–1

questions answered, your:
  milk feeding in the first year
    85–90
  sleep, understanding your baby's
    103–7
  solid food, introducing 284–90
  why follow a routine? 41–53

recommendations, important
    162–3
reflux 302–5
refusal of milk 327–8
refusal of solids 328–9
reheating tips 264
routine, why follow a? 32–53
routines, CLB and see Contented
    Little Baby (CLB) routines

salt 261–2
separation anxiety 306–9
settling your baby:
  difficulties in 334–7
  important recommendations
    162–3
Schaefer, Charles 132
sleep:
  bedtime routine 97–100
  CLB routines and see Contented
    Little Baby (CLB) routines
  daytime sleep, structuring
    during the first year 131–46
    see also sleep
  demand feeding and 94–5
  early-morning waking 100–3,
    339–41
  naps:
    importance of 132–3
    late-afternoon nap 144–6

sleep: (*continued*)
  lunch, managing sleeping and naps when going out to 151–2
  lunchtime nap 141–4, 208–9, 347–53
  splitting 137
  sleep associations 353
  problems, common sleeping 334–55
    assisting to sleep method 337–9
    breast-fed baby not settling in the evening 336–7
    early-morning waking 100–3, 339–41
    excessive night waking 342–6
    illness and 346–7
    lunchtime nap 347–53
    settling, difficulties in 334–7
    sleep associations 353
    sleep regression 354–5
    teething and night waking 353–4
  sleep required during the first year, guide to 162–3
  sleep rhythms 96–7
  sleeping routine, understanding the 133–41
  understanding your baby's 91–107
  your questions answered 103–7
Sleep: The Secret of Problem-free Nights (Beatrice Hollyer/ Lucy Smith) 319
sleepy feeder 324–6
sling, baby 15–16
snowsuit 28
socialising, guidelines for successful 155–7
socks 26
solid food, introducing 257–90
  begin, how to 265–7
  breast-fed babies 260
  early weaning 264–7
  first stage: six to seven months 267–74
    beaker, introducing a 271
    breakfast, introducing 269–70
    daily requirements 272–4
    foods to introduce 268–9
    protein at lunchtime, introducing 270–1
    tea 272
  foods to be avoided 260–2
    salt 261–2
    sugar 261
  preparing and cooking food for your baby 262–4
    defrosting tips 264
    packing food for the freezer 263
    reheating tips 264
    sterilised feeding equipment 263
  second stage: seven to nine months 274–9
    breakfast 276–7
    daily requirements 278–9
    foods to introduce 275–6
    lunch 277
    tea 278
  third stage: nine to twelve months 279–84
    breakfast 280
    daily requirements 282–4
    lunch 280–1
    tea 282
  weaning your baby 257–60
  your questions answered 284–90
sterilised feeding equipment 263
steriliser 22–3
stranger anxiety 309–10
sugar 261
swaddle, how to 26–8
Symon, Dr Brian: *Silent Nights* 323

tea 272, 278, 282
teat brush 22
teats 21
teething, night waking and 353–4

time change, helping your baby
  adjust to a different 158–9
tiredness 297–8, 334, 335, 337 *see
  also* overtiredness
tongue tie 332–4
tumble dryer, use of 30

vests 24–5

waking:
  CLB routines and waking your
    baby 42–3
  early-morning 100–3, 339–41,
    354, 357
  excessive night 342–6, 354
  teething and night 353–4
wardrobe 8
washing-up bowl 22
water, giving to babies under six
    months 83–4
weaning:
  from breast to bottle 71–3
  solid food, introducing 257–90
    see also solid food,
    introducing
weeks one to two 164–75
  changes to be made during the
    one-to two-week routine
    172–4
    feeding 173–4
    sleeping 172–3
  moving on to the two-to four
    week routine 174–5
  routine – one to two weeks
    166–72
    7am 167
    8.15am 167
    8.15/8.30am 167
    9.45am 168
    10am 168
    10.45am 168
    11/11.15am 168
    11.30am–2pm 169
    12 noon 169

2–2.30pm 169
    3.30pm 170
    5pm 170
    5.45pm 170
    6/6.15pm 170–1
    6.30/7pm 171
    8pm 171
    9.45pm 171
    10pm 171–2
    in the night 172
  starting the routine 164–6
    with premature babies 165–6
    with older babies 166
weeks two to four 176–87
  changes to be made during the
    two-to four-week routine
    182–4
    feeding 184–7
    sleeping 183–4
  routine – two to four weeks
    176–82
    7am 176–7
    8.30/8.45am 177
    9.45am 177
    10am 177
    10.30am 177
    11.15/11.30am 178
    11.45am 178
    11.30am/12 noon–2pm 178
    12/12.30pm 179
    2pm/2.30pm 179
    3.45–4pm 180
    5pm 180
    5.45pm 180
    6/6.15pm 180–1
    6.30/7pm 181
    8pm 181
    9.30pm 181
    10/10.30pm 181–2
    in the night 182
weeks four to six 188–99
  changes to be made during the
    four-to six-week routine
    194–9

weeks four to six (*continued*)
  feeding 198–9
  sleeping 194–7
  routine – four to six weeks
    188–94
    7am 188–9
    8.45am 189
    9.45am 189
    10am 189
    10.30am 189
    11.30am 190
    11.45am 190
    11.30am/12 noon–2/2.30pm
      190
    12 noon 190
    2/2.30pm 191
    4/4.15pm 191
    5pm 191–2
    5.45pm 192
    6pm 192
    6.15pm 192
    7pm 192–3
    8pm 193
    9.30pm 193
    10/10.30pm 193
    in the night 193–4
weeks six to eight 200–11
  changes to be made during six–to
    eight-week routine 207–11
  lunchtime nap 208–9
  feeding 209–11
  sleeping 207–9
  routine – six to eight weeks 200–7
    7am 200–1
    8.50am 201
    9am 201
    9.45am 201
    10am 201
    10.45am 202
    11.30am 202
    11.45am 202
    11.45am/12 noon–2/2.30pm
      202

    12 noon 203
    2/2.30pm 203
    4.15/4.30pm 204
    5pm 204
    5.45pm 204
    6pm 204
    6.15pm 205
    6.45–7pm 205
    8pm 205
    9.30pm 205
    10/10.30pm 205–6
    in the night 206–7
weeks eight to twelve 212–20
  changes to be made during
    the eight-to twelve-week
    routine 217–20
  feeding 218–19
  sleeping 217–18
moving on to the three- month
  to four-month routine 220
routine – eight to twelve weeks
    212–20
    7am 212–13
    8.50am 213
    9am 213
    9.45am 213
    10am 213
    10.45am/11am 213
    11.45am 213
    12 noon–2/2.15pm 214
    2/2.15pm 214–15
    4.15pm 215
    5pm 215
    5.45pm 215
    6pm 215
    6.15pm 216
    7pm 216
    8pm 216
    9.30pm 216
    10/10.30pm 216–17
    in the night 217
Weissbluth, Marc 132, 295–6
wind 298

Your Baby and Toddler Problems Solved

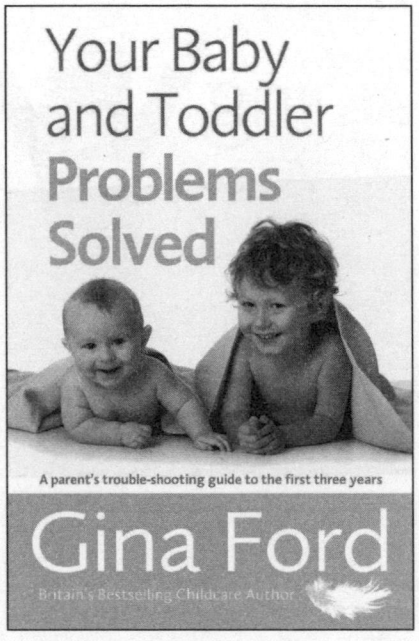

Bringing together decades of successful work with families, *Your Baby and Toddler Problems Solved* provides answers to hundreds of baby and toddler care challenges.

Organised chronologically for easy reference and with detailed case studies and examples, Gina Ford, one of the UK's bestselling childcare authors, shares her practical and realistic solutions to help you and your baby or toddler have a contented household now and for years to come.

It is Gina's belief that sleeping and feeding are intrinsically linked and that all too often babies and toddlers are subjected to unnecessary sleep training methods. Whether your baby or toddler is a fussy feeder or waking up several times a night, her holistic and gentle approach will ensure that your child's feeding and sleeping needs are fully met, and that you resolve the root cause of the problem for good.

Potty Training in One Week

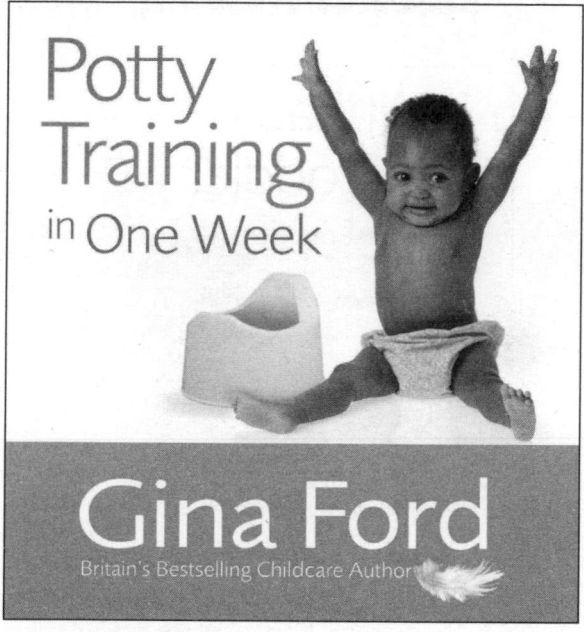

Gina Ford is the queen of routine, and one area she knows from experience that can be a big, scary hurdle for parents is potty training. The good news is that's it's very easy when you know all the tips and tricks and there is no need for tantrums or endless hours spent sitting with a toddler who refuses to go potty. This very clearly organised book answers all your questions and makes potty training easy, and even fun. You will quickly learn:

How to know when your child is really ready
How to make potty training fun for your child
How to reward
How to deal with little accidents
Why you need a potty for upstairs and for downstairs
How to help your child get over bed-wetting

With a little know-how from one of the UK's leading parenting authors, potty training will be as easy as A, B, C.

The Contented Little Baby
Book of Weaning

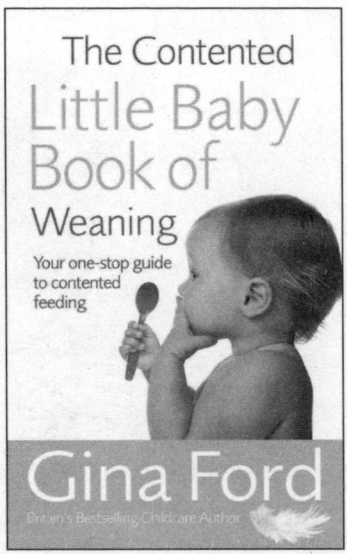

Weaning your baby on to solid foods is one of the most important milestones during the early months of parenthood, and Gina's expert advice on weaning makes a baby's transition from milk to solid foods as straightforward as possible. Successful weaning establishes a pattern of healthy eating in babies, avoiding the pitfalls of fussy eaters restricted to a narrow diet.

In this revised edition of The Contented Little Baby Book of Weaning, Gina includes the latest recommendations regarding breast-feeding and the introduction of solid food from the World Health Organisation and the UK Department of Health. She aims to take the worry out of weaning, guiding parents step-by-step through the process and shares the insight and expertise gained from personally helping to care for over 300 babies, and advising thousands more parents via her consultation service and website.

The Contented Little Baby Book of Weaning is the definitive guide to ensuring babies eat well now and as they grow up and is as relevant and helpful to those parents who have not previously followed Gina's routines.

The Contented Toddler Years

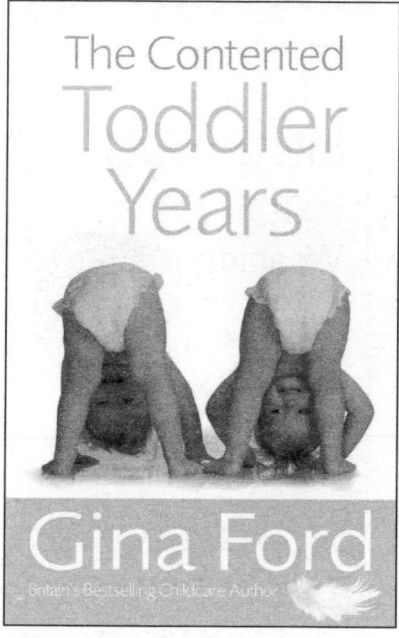

As babies grow, so their routines and patterns change. In *The Contented Toddler Years* Gina addresses the many changes in sleeping and feeding habits that arise during the second and third year. She offers invaluable advice and insight into these crucial stages of a child's development, from walking and talking, to teething and potty training and also shows you how to:

- deal with tantrums, food refusal and sibling jealousy
- prepare for the arrival of a second baby, including how to cope physically, emotionally and financially, and how to adapt her routines when caring for a baby and toddler
- make teeth-cleaning fun and put an end to habits such as thumb-sucking, nail-biting and eating dirt
- decide what type of childcare is best for you and your toddler

Reassuring and down-to-earth, parents will find Gina's advice can help make the passage from contented baby to confident child a happy and stress-free experience for the whole family.